# T H E

# *Face Book*

## A Consumer's Guide to
## Facial Plastic Surgery

**Campbell Facial Plastic Surgery**

Andrew C. Campbell, M.D.
**Facial Plastic Surgeon**
**Otolaryngologist**

**Medical Arts**
2920 Superior Avenue
Sheboygan, WI
Phone: (920) 803-FACE • Fax: (920) 459-7665
(3223)

# THE

# *Face Book*

## A Consumer's Guide to Facial Plastic Surgery

Prepared by the
American Academy
of Facial Plastic and
Reconstructive Surgery

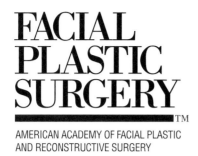

**FACIAL PLASTIC SURGERY**™
AMERICAN ACADEMY OF FACIAL PLASTIC
AND RECONSTRUCTIVE SURGERY

**Library of Congress Cataloging-in-Publication Data**
The face book: a consumer's guide to facial plastic surgery/
    American Academy of Facial Plastic and Reconstructive Surgery.
      p.     cm.
      ISBN 0-9651231-1-1 (alk. paper)
      1. Face--Surgery. 2. Surgery, Plastic. 3. Consumer education.
I. American Academy of Facial Plastic and Reconstructive Surgery.
RD119.5.F33F29 1997
617.5'20592--dc21
97-33558 CIP

**This book is available at quantity discounts with bulk purchase for educational, business, or sales promotional use. For information, contact:**
Publications Department
American Academy of Facial Plastic and Reconstructive Surgery

310 S. Henry Street
Alexandria, VA 22314
Phone: (703) 299-9291
Fax: (703) 299-8898

**Online orders:** The Face Book and other patient information materials can be ordered online at the AAFPRS web site: ***http://www.facemd.org.***

Soft cover price: $29.95 (Discounts may be available from the publisher.)

# Contents

# Facial Plastic Surgery Today

In recent years, technology has transformed the practice of facial plastic surgery. Today, surgeons can treat a wider variety of problems than ever before, and they can do so more effectively—with more natural-looking and longer-lasting results, faster healing times, and lower costs.

Consider lasers. In skillful hands, these amplified beams of light can vaporize blemishes and birthmarks once thought to be permanent. They can smooth acne scars and iron out wrinkles, and they provide surgeons with an alternative way to create a natural hairline when transplanting tiny, hair-bearing grafts to balding areas of the scalp.

Other tools and techniques allow surgeons to give the face and neck more pleasing contours. Facelifts can now tighten underlying tissue and muscles as well as skin, creating a natural look quite unlike the stretched look of earlier days. Liposuction can remove fatty deposits from areas resistant to diet and exercise. Natural and synthetic fillers can plump up deep furrows and

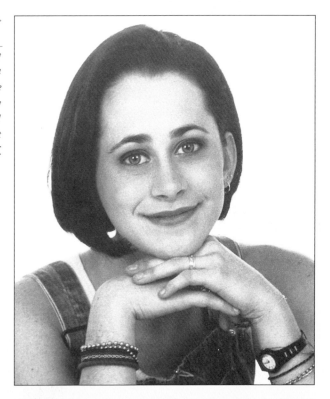

*Nasal surgery made a big difference in the way 16-year-old Jennifer felt about herself.*

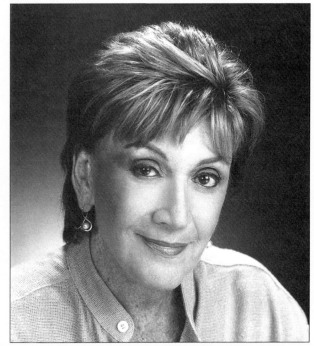

*Ronnie, who is 72, underwent facelift surgery, eyelid surgery, and full-face laser resurfacing to undo the effects of a lifetime of sun-worshiping.*

wrinkles, and a vast array of implants can give new definition to flat cheeks, receding chins, and underprojected noses.

If technology has advanced cosmetic surgery, it has produced even greater wonders for reconstructive surgery. Advances in microvascular surgery have made it possible to transplant nerves and have increased the survival of grafts and flaps used to replace damaged or destroyed skin or tissue. The amount of healthy skin available to cover an injured area can now be increased with balloon-like devices called tissue expanders. For injuries to the skeletal structure of the face, surgeons can use a variety of techniques—from building up depressions with synthetic materials to grafting bone taken from the skull, hip, or leg to an area where bone is missing or damaged beyond repair. Broken or shattered facial bones can be repaired by attaching wires to tiny screws placed in healthy bone, or by fixing metal rods or plates over the fracture, among other techniques.

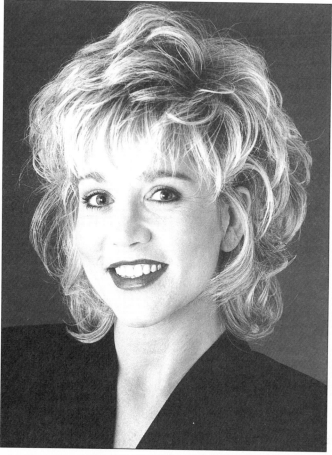

*An eyelid tuck, endoscopic browlift, and nasal procedure gave Stephanie a fresh, new look at age 33.*

It's no wonder that facial plastic surgery today is sought by a growing number of people who want to improve facial harmony, rejuvenate premature signs of aging, or repair problems present from birth or caused by accident or illness.

## THE PSYCHOLOGY OF APPEARANCE

Although techniques have changed, the goal of facial plastic surgery has not. It has remained unchanged since it was first expressed in 1931 by a German surgeon named Jacques Joseph. Generally acclaimed as the father of the modern specialty, Joseph (1865-1934) developed his theories while treating soldiers who suffered disfigurement in the trench warfare of World War I. He came to believe that people's psychological well-being depends, to large degree, on their sense of self-esteem. Self-esteem, he said, is enhanced when the facial features are in harmony. He believed that a person whose looks caused social or economic disadvantage was as severely afflicted as a person with a debilitating disease, and that the psychological outcome of aesthetic surgery was as important as its physical success.

Today, the link between physical appearance and self-esteem is widely recognized by medical professionals, who see a healthy attitude—not mere vanity—in society's emphasis on appearance.

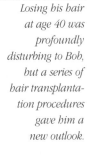

*Losing his hair at age 40 was profoundly disturbing to Bob, but a series of hair transplantation procedures gave him a new outlook.*

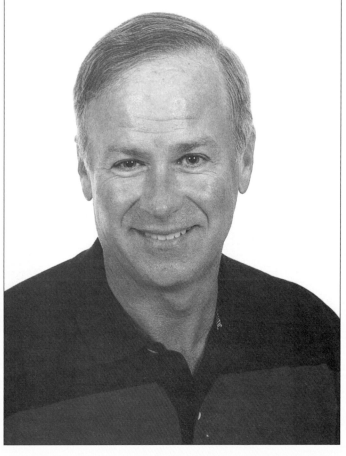

The point of looking your best, says psychologist Joyce Brothers, is to be able to forget about yourself and still exude self-confidence. "When you look good and feel great, people treat you as if you're special," she explains. "Your appearance sends signals to others about who you are, how you feel, even about your values and aspirations. When people treat you as if you are intelligent and friendly, you behave that way, and that starts an upward spiral of success."

Abigail Van Buren (Dear Abby) agrees. Looking good is a personal gift to oneself, not a narcissistic indulgence, she says. She is backed by expert psychiatric consultants, all of whom regard a little vanity as a good thing. Attention to one's looks is a sign of self-esteem, just as lack of interest in grooming and outer appearance is an early sign of depression.

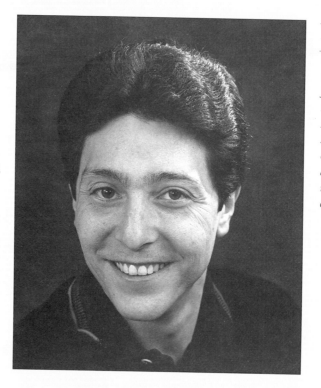

*Mugged at gunpoint and left for dead, Joe, age 30, suffered severe facial injuries. Advanced reconstructive procedures corrected the damage and helped him recover his self-confidence.*

Edward Stainbrook, former professor emeritus of psychiatry and behavioral science at the University of Southern California's School of Medicine, saw a direct link between the resurgent national interest in healthy bodies and the rise in popularity of facial plastic surgery. "If you look at the whole social cultural trend over the last 30 or 40 years, it's moving toward fitness and wellness. There is much less guilt about altering the body. To be physically well means to be physically attractive. And this affects people's willingness to use facial plastic surgery."

This link between health and appearance may well be why most people considering facial plastic surgery have very realistic expectations, according to a recent study. They desire:

- to have a tidy appearance,

  ■ to escape being regarded as different,

  ■ to have the normal physical endowments for the group to which
    they belong,

  ■ to re-establish a previously satisfactory appearance, or

  ■ to avoid being discounted as a useful member of society on
    the basis of their age.

Those people who embark on facial plastic surgery with such healthy
attitudes often come away not only looking better, but feeling good. "The physical transformation of surgery often is the catalyst that sparks renewed zest for
living," says one facial plastic surgeon. "And this secondary benefit sometimes
is far more striking than the anatomical change."

## NOT FOR EVERYONE

If you feel you might benefit from facial plastic surgery, be assured that people
all across America—from all walks of life and age groups—are opting for procedures they believe will correct a variety of problems. A number of them are
featured in this introduction, and you'll meet more in the pages to follow.

But heed this word of caution: These patients shared their stories
because facial plastic surgery helped them feel better about themselves. Facial
plastic surgery is not for everyone, and this book is not intended to suggest that
it is. A new look will not guarantee success on the job or the dating circuit. It
will not make people like you more or help a faltering marriage. What it may
do is simply make you look better, healthier, and more vibrant.

If that's what you want from facial plastic surgery, then this book
is for you. You'll get information on how to find a facial plastic surgeon and
what happens during a consultation visit. You'll learn how each procedure is
done, what the healing process is like, and what kind of results can be

achieved. You'll learn how skin type and other factors may affect the success of a facial plastic surgery procedure. And you'll get some tips on how to enhance postoperative results by following a healthful regimen—and the doctor's instructions for care.

Still interested? Then, read on. This book is your guide to facial plastic surgery today.

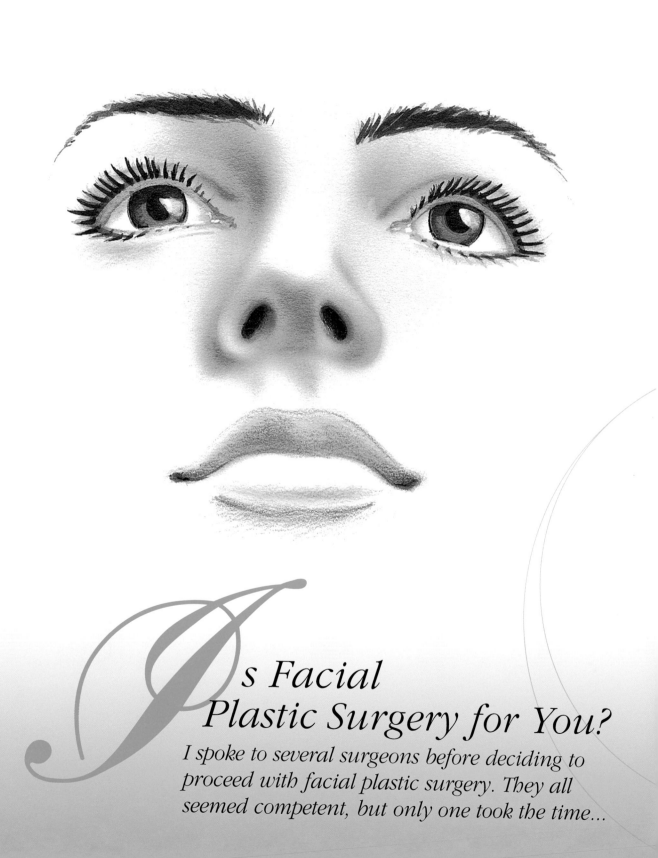

# *Is Facial Plastic Surgery for You?*

*I spoke to several surgeons before deciding to proceed with facial plastic surgery. They all seemed competent, but only one took the time…*

# *Is Facial Plastic Surgery for You?*

*"I spoke to several surgeons before deciding to proceed with facial plastic surgery. They all seemed competent, but only one really took the time to answer all my questions and make me feel comfortable. I appreciated that. You need to have a lot of trust in someone who's going to operate on your face."*

■ *Jeanine Codispotti, age 30*

■ If you're concerned about some aspect of your appearance, you should consider a consultation with a qualified facial plastic surgeon. A consultation does not commit you to a surgical procedure, but it can help you make an informed decision about surgery to achieve the improvement you desire.

## SELECTING A FACIAL PLASTIC SURGEON

Plan to do some careful research before deciding which facial plastic surgeon to consult. Should the consultation lead to surgery, your satisfaction with the results will depend on the technical expertise—and, in many cases, the artistic skill—of the person you select. You also want to find someone with whom you are comfortable and who regularly achieves good results performing the surgery you seek.

What's the best way to go about locating the surgeon who is right for you? You might start with the telephone directory, a local hospital's referral line, or even an Internet search, but don't stop there. These sources tell you little about a surgeon's abilities. A more informed source is often a friend or relative who has had facial plastic surgery.

"A surgeon's reputation always gets around," says Joan Higgins, who relied on word-of-mouth advertising to find the surgeon who performed her facelift. Pleased with the results, she's convinced that satisfied patients are the most reliable indicators of competent surgeons.

1
--------------
*A large percentage of all facial plastic and reconstructive surgery is performed by board-certified otolaryngologists, whose rigorous training in the complicated head and neck area includes extensive experience with facial plastic surgery techniques.*

Her point is a good one. However, don't base your decision entirely on just one other person's experience. Remember, every patient's needs are unique, and every surgery is different.

You might ask your family doctor for a referral. In this instance, be sure to ask how well your doctor knows not just the surgeon, but also his or her experience performing the procedure you want. Ask questions like: Have you recommended any other patients to this surgeon? What feedback have you gotten from them? Would you send a member of your family to this surgeon?

"I questioned my doctor, my wife's doctor, and every nurse we knew," recalls Bill T. "I wanted my surgery done by an expert, so I kept asking, 'Who's the best facial plastic surgeon in town?' One name popped up repeatedly, and that's the person I chose."

Not surprisingly, hair stylists often have inside information on which facial plastic surgeons patients like the most: "We hear people's stories and see the work of many facial plastic surgeons up close," says one hair stylist. Long before she decided to get her own eyes done, she already knew which surgeon did excellent eyelid surgery.

Many people like to check a surgeon's credentials before scheduling a visit. The office staff can tell you about the surgeon's specialty training, as well as the hospitals that have granted operating privileges, the medical societies in which the surgeon is active, and so forth.

The staff also can tell you which medical specialty board has certified the surgeon. Although board certification is not the only indicator of competence, it is a benchmark of excellence, indicating that a surgeon has received extensive training in a specialty and has passed an exhaustive battery of written and oral examinations.

In asking about board certification, be aware that a number of medical specialty boards test for competence in particular plastic surgery techniques—including otolaryngology/head-and-neck surgery, dermatology, ophthalmology, and general plastic surgery. Not surprisingly, a large percentage of all facial plastic and reconstructive surgery is performed by board-certified otolaryngologists, whose rigorous training in the complicated head and neck area includes extensive experience with facial plastic surgery techniques. Many otolaryngologists also are certified by the American Board of Facial Plastic and Reconstructive Surgery—the only board that sets standards, examines, and certifies surgeons exclusively in facial plastic and reconstructive surgery.

"I checked my surgeon out carefully before meeting with him," says Agnes W. "I called his office to ask questions, asked the medical society about his professional reputation, and went to the library to learn whether he had been certified by an examining board."

*Many otolaryngologists also are certified by the American Board of Facial Plastic and Reconstructive Surgery—the only board that sets standards, examines, and certifies surgeons exclusively in facial plastic and reconstructive surgery.*

## PREPARING FOR THE CONSULTATION VISIT

Once you have identified a surgeon, your next step is to schedule a visit to meet the doctor. At this point, you may not actually be ready to commit to surgery—you simply are meeting the facial plastic surgeon. Many patients interview several surgeons before making a final decision about having surgery. Although a consultation fee may be charged, the cost is well worth the satisfaction.

Ask questions, and pay attention to the surgeon's manner. Does it inspire confidence? Is he or she easy to talk to? Are all your questions answered patiently and completely? Do you feel comfortable in conversation with the surgeon?

"My doctor was so confident and professional," says Jose Nichols, a nasal surgery patient. "It was clear he knew what he was doing. That gave me confidence."

The office surroundings can provide additional insight about the surgeon. Do you see signs of a busy practice with many satisfied patients? Is the staff friendly, professional, and helpful? Does the decor convey a feeling of artistic harmony and good taste?

"I sensed that my surgeon had the soul of an artist," says Ruth Yag, who had brow and eyelid surgery. "The other doctors I interviewed didn't seem to have that artistic flair—and it showed in their photos. My surgeon's appreciation of aesthetics was important to me."

As Ruth points out, viewing before-and-after photos of the surgeon's work can help you evaluate his or her aesthetic sense and surgical skill. Photos also may help clarify what a given procedure will accomplish, as well as point out other corrections that may improve your facial harmony.

"Pictures were very important to me," says Julie Kern, who sought surgery to repair a nasal problem. "Some doctors made promises but couldn't show me any pictures. When I found a surgeon who showed me photos of people with problems like mine that demonstrated how he had treated them, I knew he could do what he said he would."

To help you prepare for your consultation, you may ask the doctor to send you information on the type of surgery that interests you. Many surgeons are happy to send you brochures that describe the procedures they perform and that provide other useful information.

Terri Speck found this step to be invaluable in preparing for her consultation. "The doctor sent me a lot of literature to read about facial resurfacing," she recounts. "This made me aware of the different options, and helped me think of the questions I needed to ask when I sat down with him."

*Good candidates for facial plastic surgery understand how facial plastic surgery can improve their appearance, but they are not looking for perfection.*

## THE AGING PROCESS

Although several factors play a role in determining how rapidly your face shows the effects of age, each decade is associated with certain changes. Your surgeon will evaluate your face to determine the extent of these changes and recommend appropriate corrective procedures. The following chart lists typical changes for each decade and refers you to the chapter of this book that describes how the problem may be treated. You may want to use it to prepare for your consultation visit.

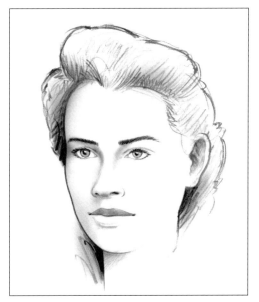

◀ *Figure 1*

# Age 30

| Typical changes | Corrective procedures |
| --- | --- |
| Upper eyelids begin to droop; pouches form in the lower lids | Eyelid surgery, *see Chapter 4* |
| Fine lines appear under the eyes | Skin resurfacing, *see Chapter 9* |
| Frown lines form in brow area | Browlift, *see Chapter 5* |
| Wrinkles appear around mouth | Injectable fillers, *see Chapter 2* Skin resurfacing, *see Chapter 9* |

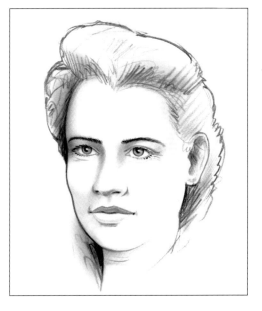

◀ *Figure 2*

# Age 40

| Typical changes | Corrective procedures |
| --- | --- |
| Upper and lower eyelids start to sag; crow's feet appear | Eyelid surgery, *see Chapter 4* Skin resurfacing, *see Chapter 9* |
| Frown lines in brow deepen; horizontal wrinkles appear | Browlift, *see Chapter 5* |
| Vertical lines around lips deepen; wrinkles become more prominent | Injectable fillers, *see Chapter 2* Skin resurfacing, *see Chapter 9* |
| In some men, male pattern baldness may be evident | Hair grafts or scalp flap surgery, *see Chapter 8* |

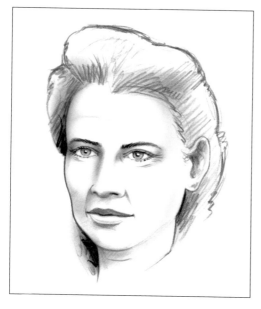

◀ *Figure 3*

# Age 50

| Typical changes | Corrective procedures |
| --- | --- |
| Pouches become prominent in the upper cheek area | Eyelid surgery, *see Chapter 4* <br> Cheek implant, *see Chapter 6* |
| Double chin develops | Facelift, liposuction, *see Chapter 2* |
| Eyebrows sag; deeper horizontal lines appear in brow | Browlift, *see Chapter 5* |
| Jaw line sags and jowls form | Facelift, *see Chapter 2* |
| Nasal tip begins to droop | Nasal surgery, *see Chapter 3* |

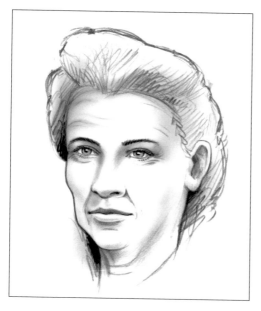

◀ *Figure 4*

# Age 60+

| Typical changes | Corrective procedures |
| --- | --- |
| Eyelids develop a distinct hooded appearance | Eyelid surgery, *see Chapter 4* |
| The facial skin loses its elasticity, causing the skin to sag | Facelift, *see Chapter 2* |
| Forehead lines deepen | Browlift, *see Chapter 5* |
| Deep vertical wrinkles appear around lips | Injectable fillers, *see Chapter 2* <br> Skin resurfacing, *see Chapter 9* |
| Neck skin droops and cords develop, causing "turkey wattle" | Facelift, *see Chapter 2* |

## EVALUATING YOUR MOTIVES

When you first meet with the surgeon, you should explain exactly what you think is wrong with your face and what you would like the surgery to accomplish. Be straightforward and specific. Although the problem may seem obvious to you, don't be surprised if the doctor asks you to describe it in detail and tell why you want to make a change.

Be prepared to answer questions like: Why do you want to correct this problem? What do you expect the surgery to do for you? Has anyone else urged you to have surgery? What is your goal in seeking this change?

# *What constitutes attractiveness?*

Beauty—despite the old adage—is much more than skin deep. In fact, in a real sense, facial attractiveness is largely determined by what lies beneath the skin—the contours and dimensions of the underlying bone structure.

Facial plastic surgeons are trained to recognize the skeletal proportions that determine attractiveness. For this reason, your surgeon will analyze your bone structure and facial features carefully before discussing any possible improvements, perhaps using aesthetic principles similar to these:

*Figure 5*
*Rule of thirds*
*and fifths*

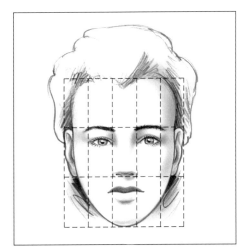

A key principle of facial proportion is based on the "golden proportion," a concept that has long been recognized in architecture and art. It states that a well proportioned face will be divided into equal thirds when horizontal lines are drawn through the forehead hairline, the brow, the base of the nose, and the edge of the chin *(see Figure 5)*.

A proportionate face may be divided vertically into fifths, each approximately the width of one eye. Aesthetic balance is considered ideal when the facial features fall within these parameters *(see Figure 5)*.

*Figure 6*
*Facial*
*symmetry*

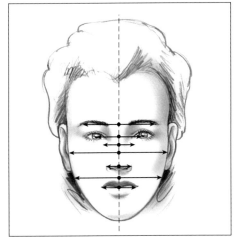

Although small differences contribute to individuality, an attractive face exhibits a high degree of bilateral symmetry, that is, similarity between one side of the face and the other *(see Figure 6)*.

It was once widely believed that standards of beauty were largely cultural. New research suggests, however, that our views of what is attractive are remarkably consistent, regardless of race, nationality, or age. Although the preference for individual features may vary among cultures, the proportions of facial attractiveness are generally the same for most ethnic groups.

Aesthetic principles are helpful, but they are only a guideline. People today appreciate individual uniqueness, and they know that true beauty starts from within.

The surgeon will probe thoroughly into your attitudes regarding surgery because realistic expectations are crucial to success. Good candidates for facial plastic surgery understand how facial plastic surgery can improve their appearance, but they are not looking for perfection. They are strongly motivated and understand that surgery involves a certain amount of discomfort and weeks—perhaps months—of swelling or discoloration.

Individuals with unrealistic expectations, on the other hand, are likely to be disappointed with even the best of surgical results. For this reason, surgeons are hesitant to operate on people with peculiar reasons for wanting surgery, those who are seeking more than surgery can do, and those who are being pressured into the surgery by someone else.

Bring in pictures of faces you like, as well as ones you do not like, in order to communicate your desires more clearly to the surgeon. Remember, however, that pictures are only a tool. Facial plastic surgery is highly individualized, and no procedure gives an identical result in every patient. The goal of surgery is to improve and harmonize your unique features, not to put someone else's features on your face. Don't bring in a picture and tell the surgeon, "Make me look like this," or "I want a nose exactly like this one." Doing so may indicate that you don't really understand what facial plastic surgery is all about—and the surgeon may well conclude that you are not a good candidate for surgery.

## VISUALIZING THE RESULTS

It's natural, when you are planning a facial plastic surgery procedure, to wonder what you will look like afterward. No one can show you an exact picture of your "new face," but facial plastic surgeons have a variety of ways to help you visualize your appearance after surgery.

The simplest way is to view before-and-after photos of patients who have had a similar procedure. Although this doesn't show how you will look, it can give you insight into the surgeon's aesthetic taste.

"I worried that eyelid surgery would give me an unnatural, wide-eyed appearance. The photos proved my fears were groundless," one patient notes. Says another, "After seeing a number of pictures, I knew I could put myself in the doctor's hands and trust him to give me a nose that looked right for my face."

Some surgeons may sketch the proposed correction—to a nose or chin, for instance—directly onto a photograph taken of your face during the consultation. Others may make a sketch of your face showing the proposed improvement.

Many surgeons use a quick and easy way to show what a facelift or browlift might do for you: Simply place your thumbs on your temples and your fingertips at your hairline and lift upward and backward while looking into a mirror. The improvement you see shows approximately what you can expect.

*Your surgical outcome depends on many factors, including your underlying bone structure, the quality of your cartilage, the texture of your skin, and your personal healing capacity.*

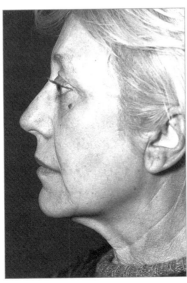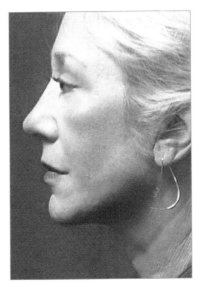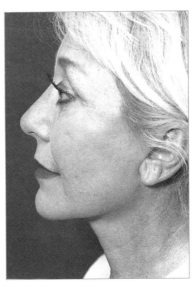

▲ *Computer imaging is one way facial plastic surgeons help patients visualize their appearance after surgery. This woman's photos—(l. to r.) actual photo before surgery; computer-generated postoperative photo; and actual photo after surgery—show postoperative results that closely resemble those projected with computer imaging.*

A more high-tech approach is computer imaging. The surgeon may photograph your face with a video camera and transfer the image to a high-resolution monitor. A computer input device then is used to manipulate the image, showing you what you might look like after the procedure. Remember, though, that computer imaging is intended only to help you visualize a proposed change. It cannot predict actual surgical results.

Your surgical outcome depends on many factors, including your underlying bone structure, the quality of your cartilage, the texture of your skin, and your personal healing capacity. Remember, too, that it takes several weeks or months to see the final results. Although much of the healing takes place within two weeks after surgery, subtle improvement may continue for up to one year.

## FORMULATING A TREATMENT PLAN

After discussing your concerns, the surgeon will evaluate your face, examining your skin texture and bone structure and taking measurements of your facial features. Medical photographs of your face will be taken, probably from several angles. These are used by the surgeon in planning your procedure. (You may be asked to sign a release form, allowing the photos to be used for educational or other purposes.)

Keep an open mind. Even if you know exactly what procedure you need, don't be surprised if the surgeon suggests an alternative plan. Facial plastic surgeons are skilled in evaluating facial harmony and suggesting procedures to give optimal results.

"I thought I needed nose surgery," explains Gloria M. "The doctor helped me to see that premature signs of aging were more of a problem." Gloria opted for eyelid surgery, liposuction, and a chemical peel. "I'm absolutely thrilled with the results," she says. "I'm going back soon for a chin implant, which will give my face balance and make my nose less prominent."

The surgeon also will take a careful medical history. To ensure the best possible surgical outcome, you should be completely candid regarding such factors as your smoking history, use of drugs and medications (including aspirin and other over-the-counter pain relievers), alcohol consumption, and past evidence of a tendency to scar.

You should feel comfortable with every aspect of the proposed treatment plan and have a clear understanding of what to expect. Take your time, ask questions, and be sure you understand everything. Don't forget to ask about the practical aspects of the procedure, such as the cost, payment arrangements, and insurance coverage.

It may help to bring a close friend or trusted family member to the consultation visit. A supportive friend can help you relax, remind you of questions to ask, and help you remember details of the discussion later. Remember, though, that it's your consultation visit. Do not allow the other person to monopolize the conversation. You may want to discuss the proposed treatment with your spouse or a close friend before making a final decision, but do not allow anyone to rush you into making a decision.

There is nothing wrong with having two or even three consultation visits before scheduling surgery, if you find it helpful.

When Ruth Yag consulted a surgeon about a drooping eyelid, he advised her to consider a browlift as well. "I was so overwhelmed I honestly didn't know what to ask," she recalls. "He invited me to come back for a second consultation, and I returned with a whole list of questions. That gave me a better understanding of the procedure, and I appreciated his patience."

Once you and the surgeon have agreed on a treatment plan, you will be asked to sign an informed consent agreement. This indicates to the surgeon that you understand the proposed procedure and its alternatives, risks, and potential outcomes, and that you would like to have it carried out. Finally, your procedure will be scheduled, and you will be given instructions on how to prepare for surgery.

# The effect of skin type

Your facial plastic surgeon will carefully assess your skin type, because the outcome of your procedure may be affected by such factors as the thickness of your skin, the amount of oil it contains, the degree of pigmentation, and the quality of underlying cartilage. While skin type won't necessarily disqualify you for facial plastic surgery, it may be necessary to modify, or even avoid, certain procedures to minimize the possibility of scarring or prevent undesirable changes in pigmentation.

Facial plastic surgeons have identified seven basic skin types, each associated with characteristic benefits and challenges related to facial plastic surgery:

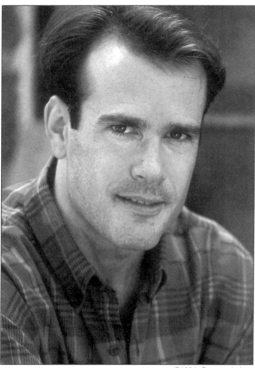

©1994, Comstock, Inc.

## Type 1—Fair, dry, thin-skinned complexion (Anglo-Saxon)

### Benefits
- Thin skin drapes easily and allows more refined results.
- Scars tend to be thin and heal well.
- Postoperative swelling is minimal.

### Challenges
- Signs of aging appear early.
- Initial bruising is more obvious than in darker skinned individuals.
- Fine, deep wrinkles may be difficult to remove entirely.
- Thin skin makes bone and cartilage irregularities more obvious.

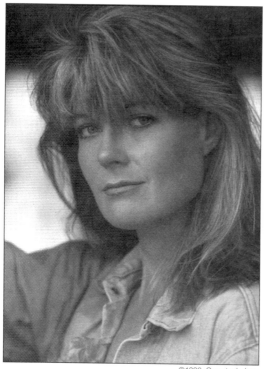

©1990, Comstock, Inc.

## Type 2—Fair, blue-eyed, blond complexion (Northern European)

### Benefits

- Skin is relatively thin and handles easily.
- Scars tend to be narrow and nearly invisible.

### Challenges

- Signs of aging appear early.
- Fine, deep wrinkles may be difficult to remove entirely.
- Initial bruising is more obvious than in darker skinned individuals.

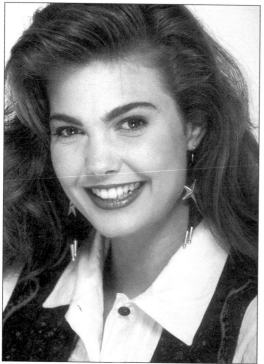

©1995, Comstock, Inc.

## Type 3—Ruddy, freckled complexion (redhead)

### Benefits

- Signs of aging appear later.
- Bone and cartilage structure usually is good.
- Scars usually are thin.

### Challenges

- Postoperative pigmentation problems may occur.
- Skin tends to bruise easily and postoperative swelling may last longer.
- Fine, white scar lines may contrast with peach skin tone.
- Skin cancers are most common in this group.

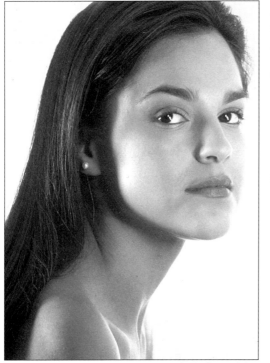

©1997, Comstock, Inc.

## Type 4—Dark, oily brunette complexion (Southern European)

### Benefits
- Signs of aging appear later.
- Fine wrinkling over entire face is less common.
- Skin cancers are less common than in lighter toned skin types.

### Challenges
- Heavier skin tends to resist lifting.
- Postoperative swelling and bruising tend to last considerably longer.
- Scars may be thicker and darker.

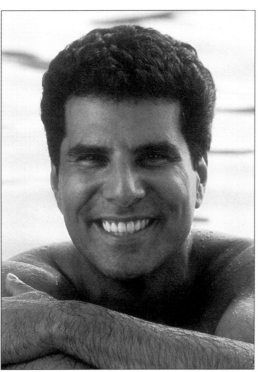

©1996, Comstock, Inc.

## Type 5—Oily, olive, dark complexion (Southern Mediterranean)

### Benefits
- Signs of aging appear later.
- Skin cancers are very rare.

### Challenges
- Darker, thicker scars are more common.
- Cartilage tends to droop and is resistant to change.
- Postoperative swelling and oiliness may be prolonged.

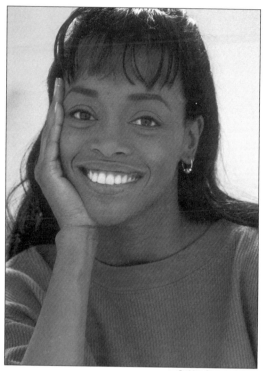

©1997, Comstock, Inc.

## Type 6—African-American complexion

### Benefits

- Signs of aging appear very late.
- Fine wrinkling typically does not occur.
- Skin cancers are very rare.
- Postoperative swelling is minimal.

### Challenges

- Formation of keloids (excessive scar growth) is possible.
- Dark or light pigmentation changes may occur.
- Thicker cartilage is not easily adjusted.

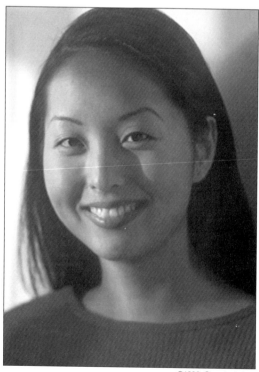

©1996, Comstock, Inc.

## Type 7—Asian complexion

### Benefits

- Signs of aging appear late.
- Fine wrinkling typically does not occur.

### Challenges

- Low nasal bridge may require correction.
- Additional surgical steps are needed to create an eyelid crease.

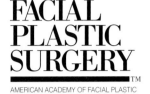

## Facial surgery on-line

Be sure to visit the Web site of the American Academy of Facial Plastic and Reconstructive Surgery. The address is:
**http://www.facemd.org.**

# What does facial plastic surgery cost?

A discussion of the cost is an important part of your consultation visit. Because insurance companies, as a rule, do not cover procedures intended solely to provide an aesthetic benefit, most facial plastic surgeons expect you to pay the cost in advance of surgery. You should ask for a written estimate of the charges, and arrange your financing before committing to the surgery.

Insurance may cover all or a portion of the charge for a procedure intended to improve function, relieve symptoms, correct a birth defect, or repair an injury. It is your responsibility to check with your insurance company and, if appropriate, arrange for reimbursement.

Be sure you understand exactly what is covered by the fee quoted. Some doctors offer a package price that includes the surgeon's fee, the charge for use of the surgical facility, and the cost of anesthesia and other medications. Other surgeons bill each item separately. Ask what is included in the cost so there will be no misunderstanding.

The fee is determined largely by the extent of the surgery, as well as the skill and training of the surgeon. Geographic location also plays a role—fees tend to be highest in New York, California, and Florida. The type of anesthesia used, the amount of follow-up needed, and whether the surgery takes place in a hospital or the surgeon's office facility are other factors that may affect the overall cost.

The following list is intended to give you an idea of the range of costs (surgeon's fee only) for some popular aesthetic procedures:

| | |
|---|---|
| *Facelift* | *$ 4,000 – $ 8,000* |
| *Nasal surgery* | *$ 3,000 – $ 7,500* |
| *Eyelid surgery* | *$ 2,500 – $ 6,000* |
| *Browlift* | *$ 1,000 – $ 4,000* |
| *Chin surgery* | *$ 500 – $ 2,000* |
| *Cheek surgery* | *$ 1,500 – $ 2,500* |
| *Ear surgery* | *$ 1,000 – $ 4,500* |
| *Hair grafting (per session)* | *$ 3,000 – $ 7,000* |
| *Scalp flap surgery* | *$10,000 – $20,000* |
| *Facial liposuction* | *$ 500 – $ 2,000* |
| *Skin resurfacing* | *$ 1,000 – $ 4,500* |

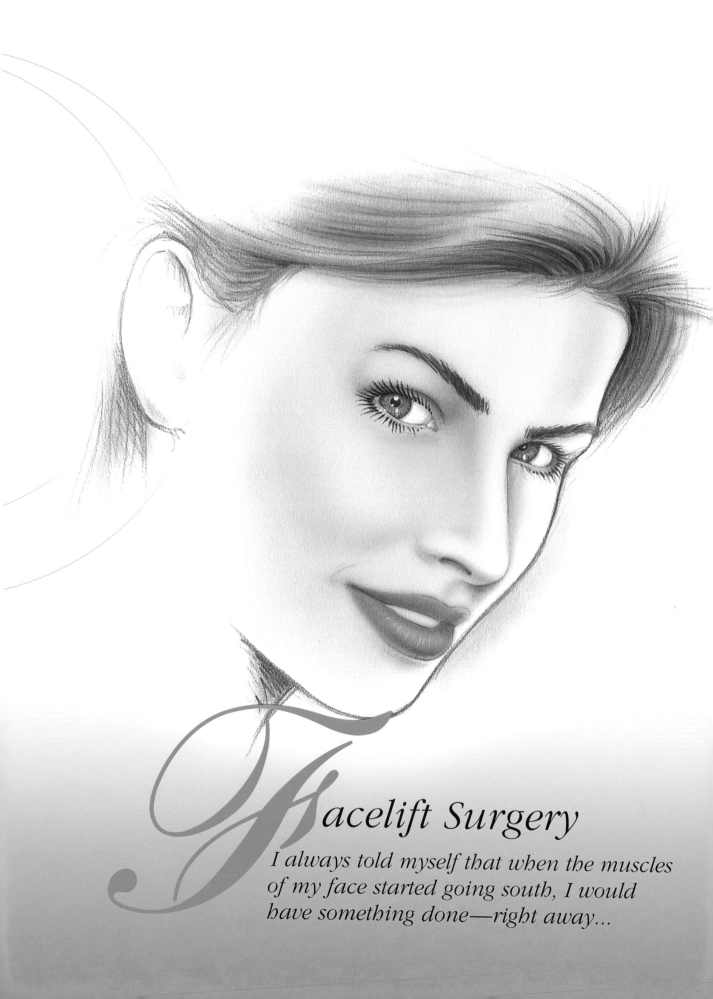

# Facelift Surgery

*I always told myself that when the muscles of my face started going south, I would have something done—right away...*

# Facelift Surgery

*"I always told myself that when the muscles of my face started going south, I would have something done—right away. I didn't want to wait so long that surgery would cause a remarkable difference. So, two months ago, I had my facelift, and I haven't regretted it for a moment. It didn't give me a new face—it gave me back my old face, the way it was 10 years ago. The changes were so subtle that no one has any idea I did it, and that's what I wanted—to look like me, only better."*

■ *Karen A., age 44*

None of us can escape the ravages of time. Inevitably, gravity, the elements, and nature take their toll. Your skin begins losing its elasticity and begins to sag. As muscles and other soft tissues weaken, jowls form along your jaw line. Smile lines become permanent, and creases develop around your mouth and chin. Your skin begins to feel too large for your face. You may begin to feel, as Karen did, that your face is "headed south."

In the past, many people were inclined to accept such changes as the cost of growing older. Today, a growing number of women—and men—are taking the attitude that there's no good reason to look older than you feel.

"I take care of myself, and I like looking good," says David D., who had a facelift at age 61. "Why live with wrinkles if I don't have to? Guys who've done this are all around," he adds with a chuckle. "Maybe they're just less likely to talk about it."

Facelift surgery is one of the most common procedures for reducing the signs of aging. Designed to lift and tighten sagging primarily in the lower part of the face, it smoothes the neck area, reduces jowls, and refines the jaw line. In younger patients, who are just beginning to notice sagging in the lower face, a facelift alone is sufficient to solve the problem. This was the case with Julie W., who had a facelift in her late 40s.

2

*Today, a growing number of women—and men—are taking the attitude that there's no good reason to look older than you feel.*

"I had some sagging in my neck area, and jowls were beginning to form," she explains. "Also, I had some deep lines beside my mouth that I wanted tightened up. The facelift made a big difference. I look much better now."

A simple facelift was ideal for Julie. You should understand, however, that a facelift alone will not improve the eyelids or eyebrows, nor will it reduce horizontal forehead wrinkles or vertical creases between the brows or around the lips. If problems such as these are evident, you may be advised to have a facelift in combination with other facial plastic surgery procedures, such as eyelid surgery, browlift, and skin resurfacing. This was Karen's experience.

"Heavy eyebrows run in my family," she explains. "The surgeon pointed out that correcting my jowls would call more attention to my permanent frown. He advised doing a browlift and facelift at the same time, and also suggested an additional procedure to remove excess fat from under my chin."

Should you have a basic facelift or a more comprehensive procedure? The choice is up to you. Discuss your concerns and expectations with your facial plastic surgeon, who will evaluate your face and suggest the facial rejuvenation procedures that can meet your specific needs.

## TOO YOUNG FOR A FACELIFT?

There is no one age that is considered ideal for a facelift. You may be in your late 30s or your upper 70s—or anywhere in between—and still be a good candidate for surgery, as long as you are in good health.

The trend in facelifts today is to have surgery at a younger age. Like Karen and Julie, many people are choosing to have corrective procedures done early, before the signs of aging have become very pronounced. In the past, the typical facelift patient was a woman in her upper 50s or early 60s with a significant amount of sagging and excess tissue in her lower face and neck areas. Today, the typical patient is likely to be in her 40s or 50s, and she may be just beginning to see some signs of aging.

Naturally, the results of a facelift in your 40s are much more subtle than they would be if you waited until the problem becomes severe. Nonetheless, there are some good reasons for having a facelift in your younger years. One is that people are less likely to notice that you have had surgery.

"I didn't want the surgery to cause a remarkable difference," notes Julie. "In fact, I didn't want people to know at all. As it turned out, the changes were very subtle. I can tell the difference, but no one else can."

Another benefit is that the procedure is somewhat shorter and simpler than it would be if you waited until the problems were more severe. You may have significantly less bruising and swelling, and you may get back to work in as few as seven to 10 days.

Although the results of an early facelift are more subtle, they seem to last a long time. This may be because the facelift creates a sheet of scar tissue in the layer of supportive tissue beneath the skin. The scar tissue is firm and stable; it holds the muscles and skin in place and prevents further slipping of the fatty tissue. Thus, an early facelift may actually seem to slow down the aging process.

On the other hand, if you are in good health, it's possible to have a facelift done at any age. Grace B. recently had a facelift at the age of 70.

"It was not difficult," she relates. "I had a lot of swelling, and I looked terrible for about a week, but it definitely was worth it. I'm glad to be rid of the jowls and the 'turkey neck.' Actually, it was a great adventure!"

## HOW A FACELIFT IS DONE

The incision for a facelift usually begins in the temple area and continues around and behind each ear. In women, the scars are usually hidden in the scalp and the natural creases of the ear *(see Figure 1)*. The incision line is modified somewhat in men to avoid unnatural patterns of beard growth or visible scarring *(see Figure 2)*.

After making the incision, the surgeon raises the skin of the temples, cheeks, and neck. The underlying connective tissue is lifted and repositioned, and permanent sutures may be placed to hold it in the new position. Excess fat and skin are removed, then the skin is redraped and the incisions are closed with sutures and small metal clips. The surgery is done without shaving or clipping any hair from the incision site.

Depending on the extent of the surgery, the procedure may take between two and four hours. It typically is done in an ambulatory surgical center or the doctor's office surgery facility, and most patients go home the same day. In some cases, an overnight hospital stay may be recommended.

Generally, facelift surgery may be done under twilight anesthesia. This involves medication given orally and intravenously, along with a local anesthetic, to keep you in a state known as "twilight sleep."

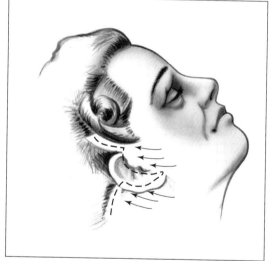

◄

*Figure 1*

*The hair and creases of the outer ear are used to hide facelift scars in women. The incision begins in the hair behind the temple, passes just within the ear, and then loops around it.*

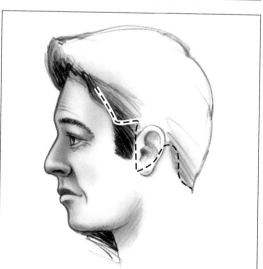

◄

*Figure 2*

*In men, the facelift incision may pass in front of each ear where it can be hidden by the sideburns. It does not pass through the ear, as in women, because that would cause beard growth in the ear.*

# More than skin deep

In earlier days, facelift surgery involved simply lifting and tightening the sagging skin of the face. Today, surgeons go deeper to tighten the supportive tissue that lies beneath the skin. That is why modern facelifts yield better, more natural-looking results.

In reality, it is not simply the skin that stretches and sags with age. The underlying tissue also is affected, and it is this deeper layer that causes much of the sagging that is associated with age. Surgeons call this layer the SMAS—short for "superficial musculoaponeurotic system." The SMAS layer forms a sort of boundary at which the superficial layers of the skin come together with the deeper muscles of the face.

To treat sagging in the underlying tissue, the surgeon elevates the SMAS layer, tightens it, and removes excess tissue. Permanent sutures may be placed in the SMAS tissue to fix it in its new position. The retaining stitches in the SMAS layer minimize tension on the skin, allowing rapid healing of the incisions with minimal scarring. Because the deeper structures are tightened as well as the surface skin, the face looks smooth and natural—without the unnatural "pulled" look that characterized some earlier facelifts.

When significant sagging has occurred in the midface region, the standard SMAS facelift may not be adequate to solve the problem. In this case, the surgeon may use a more involved technique called a deep-plane facelift.

To perform a deep-plane facelift, the surgeon elevates facial muscles and fat that lie below the SMAS layer. The fat pads of the cheek and midface, which often slip downward with age, are

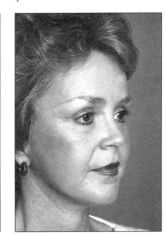

*Today's deeper facelift procedures more effectively treat the deep creases that develop between the nose and the mouth as we age.*

restored to their natural position, creating a more youthful facial contour. Because the procedure is more complex than a standard SMAS facelift, the risk of complications is somewhat higher, and bruising and swelling may be more extensive and take longer to resolve.

On the other hand, the deep-plane facelift allows more facial sculpturing to correct problems in the cheek and midface region. It is the only type of facelift procedure that may improve the deep creases that often develop on either side of the face between the nose and mouth—what doctors call nasolabial folds.

If you are concerned with problems in the midface region, your facial plastic surgeon will advise you on whether or not you may be a candidate for a deeper facelift procedure.

Although it is not as deep as general anesthesia, you will not feel pain and probably will remember nothing afterward. Depending on your preference, you may have general anesthesia or milder sedatives combined with local anesthesia to keep you relaxed and free from pain.

Julie has no memory of her facelift. "I was apprehensive, but it really was fine," she recalls. "I went to the doctor's office early in the morning, had the surgery, stayed for a short recovery period, then went home that afternoon. Afterward, I had some pain, but it was not excessive and I had medication to relieve it."

Karen was more nervous about the sedation than the surgery. "I didn't want general anesthesia, because I always get sick when I am put to sleep," she explains. "During the procedure, I wasn't exactly asleep, but I was completely detached from what was happening. I had no fear or pain at any time."

## TIGHTENING MUSCLES IN THE NECK

Correcting problems in the neck area is an important part of the facelift procedure. Although the conventional facelift smoothes and tightens the skin of the neck, it does not address weakness in the underlying muscles. An additional step sometimes is carried out to tighten these muscles.

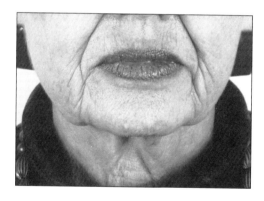 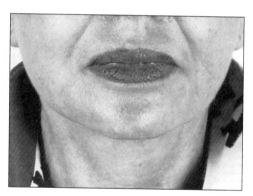

*A facelift may greatly reduce jowling and excess skin in the neck area. Here, the smoother skin and the reduction of laugh lines around the mouth are the result of a facelift and chemical peeling.*

As we age, the muscles supporting the neck—called the platysma—begin to weaken. The midline of the neck may take on a sunken appearance, with prominent vertical bands visible on either side. In some people, excess skin and fatty tissue may collect under the chin as well, forming loose deposits of hanging tissue that resemble turkey wattles.

To reach the platysmal muscles, the surgeon makes a small incision under the chin. Through this incision, the edges of the platysmal muscles are located and drawn together, then stitched together at the midline. Next, the back portion of these sheet-like muscles is tightened and fixed at the back of the neck on either side. This forms a strong sling of muscle that supports the entire neck and jaw.

Excess fatty tissue and "turkey wattles" may be removed at the same time. If necessary, lipo-suction can be done through the same incision.

Once stitched together, the platysmal muscles are less prone to sagging. For this reason, many surgeons recommend performing this step in every facelift procedure, even if the sunken effect is not yet evident.

Julie's facelift included this procedure. "I was not supposed to turn my head for the first few weeks, to give the muscles a chance to heal," she recalls. "It was worth the small inconvenience though. My neck looks fabulous, and I'm thrilled to know it will last a long time."

## AFTER THE PROCEDURE

After the surgery, a soft dressing may be placed around your head to protect the incisions. This probably will be removed within a day or so, but smaller bandages may be used for several days afterward. All dressings usually are removed within three to four days, and you are then allowed to shower and shampoo your hair. Some stitches may be removed during the first week, but staples may be left in your scalp for seven to 10 days.

Most people report little pain after facelift surgery. David D. took pain medication for the first few days, although he says the recovery process was not especially painful. Reports Julie: "There was some pain, but nothing severe. I was just uncomfortable and very anxious to get the bandage taken off."

Some swelling and bruising are to be expected after a facelift, but much of it will diminish within the first week or two. Most people are able to return to work about two weeks after surgery, although you will be advised not to do anything strenuous for at least a month. Incision lines will appear pink at first, but they can be covered with makeup as soon as they have healed. By three to four weeks after surgery, most of the healing is complete. Scars will continue to fade over the course of a year.

"I stayed in the first week, and I wore turtlenecks when I first started going out in public," says Grace B., who returned to a normal routine about 10 days after surgery.

Karen, whose procedure was much more involved, avoided going out in public for nearly three weeks. "I looked hammered," she laughs. "People who saw me thought I had been in an accident."

Your surgeon will give you detailed instructions for caring for your face after surgery. "I had to clean the incisions daily and apply a medicated ointment," explains Julie. "I got a lot of rest the first week, and I kept my head elevated to help minimize swelling. I followed all instructions to the letter, and I think it made a big difference."

Don't be surprised if you feel somewhat let down after surgery. It's not uncommon for facelift patients to experience some doubts in the week or two after surgery. "I looked so horrible, I feared I would never look normal again," Karen recalls. "I even found myself becoming weepy at times. My doctor was very reassuring, and the sad feelings soon lifted. Now I'm just delighted I did it."

# Managing fatty deposits

Fatty deposits in the neck area can be improved at the same time as a facelift by means of a procedure called liposuction. Appropriate for men and women of all ages, liposuction reduces the number of fat cells in a localized area. Although it is not recommended for persons whose excess facial fat is part of an overall weight problem, the procedure is ideal for refining the contour of the neck and jaw line and eliminating heavy jowls.

Liposuction often is done at the same time as a facelift to remove sagging fatty tissue that has collected in the lower face and neck area. It also may be done alone or in conjunction with other procedures, such as nose or chin surgery, cheek augmentation, or blepharoplasty.

To perform facial liposuction, the surgeon makes a tiny incision, usually beneath the chin or in the crease under the ears. A narrow tube called a cannula is inserted through the incision and excess fat cells are vacuumed out.

A variation of the procedure, called tumescent liposuction, involves injecting the area to be treated with a large amount of sterile salt solution in order to make it "tumescent," or firm. The saline solution contains a local anesthetic and a drug to constrict blood vessels, which may reduce discomfort and lessen the bruising that sometimes follows liposuction. The fat cells and the saline solution are vacuumed out at the same time.

After liposuction, a snug dressing is applied around the treated area. This usually is removed in the surgeon's office the next day, but you may be advised to wear a compression bandage for a few days and for several weeks at night to speed the healing of the treated area.

Most people are able to return to work a few days after having liposuction alone. If you have another procedure at the same time, you probably will not notice any additional discomfort from the liposuction. If necessary, mild pain relievers may be taken for a day or two, and ice may be applied to minimize swelling.

*Liposuction often is done at the same time as a facelift to remove sagging fatty tissue that has collected in the lower face and neck area.*

# *"The best thing I ever did"*

"The whole thing was a very positive experience," says Joan Higgins four months after she had a facelift—her second—and laser resurfacing around her mouth. "I'm absolutely thrilled with the way it turned out. When I look in the mirror, it just blows me away."

Joan had her first facelift at age 50. "A lot has changed in 20 years," she says. "It was so much easier than I remember—and this time I went home the same day."

Loose skin under her chin and vertical lines around her lips were Joan's major concerns when she sought a facial plastic surgeon's advice. "The doctor described how he could join the muscles in my neck," she explains. He showed me a photo of an 80-year-old woman who had had the procedure, and she looked wonderful. I said, 'Let's do it!' "

The whole experience was "really, truly painless," Joan maintains. "I never even took a pain pill. I just took it easy and enjoyed a good book for about 10 days. During that time, though, I was up and around, doing things for myself and getting meals for my husband."

Joan sought advice from a cosmetologist before attending a family wedding several weeks after the surgery. "Everyone commented on how nice I looked," she smiles, "but no one suspected I had surgery."

The procedure brightened both Joan's appearance and her spirits. "My husband thinks I look great," she enthuses. "He's younger than me by a few years, but I look like the younger one now. This is the best thing I ever did!"

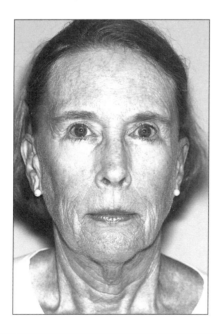 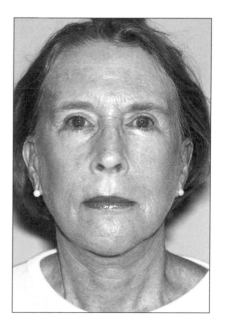

# Filling depressions and deep wrinkles

Sometimes, deep wrinkles are treated with special filler materials. This may be done as a separate procedure, or in conjunction with a facelift or other facial rejuvenation surgery.

The most commonly used injectable fillers are collagen and fat. Collagen, a gel-like substance derived from purified animal tissue, generally is used to fill out deep facial wrinkles, creases and furrows, sunken cheeks, skin depressions, and certain scars. Fat cells harvested from another part of your body, such as the abdomen or thigh area, may be used to plump up sunken cheeks; minimize forehead wrinkles, smile lines, and other deep skin depressions; or enhance the lips.

Other substances that are sometimes used as fillers include a gelatin powder compound that is mixed with your blood and injected under the skin and a thread-like synthetic material that may be implanted beneath the skin to provide support and fill deep depressions.

Injectable fillers are eventually absorbed, so the improvement they provide is temporary. Typically, the injections need to be repeated once or twice a year to maintain the correction. Occasionally, injectable fillers are used to provide a temporary improvement while a patient is considering a more permanent facial contouring procedure. Synthetic implants remain in the body indefinitely and provide a permanent solution.

Injections of fat or collagen usually are administered in a surgeon's office-based facility. No anesthetic normally is needed for collagen injections, since a numbing agent is added to the collagen itself. If you are having fat injections, both the donor and the recipient sites will be numbed with local anesthesia, or you may choose to have light sedation. After treatment, you may experience some minor stinging or throbbing in the injected area. You may look somewhat swollen for a week or so, because it is necessary to "overfill" the area slightly to compensate for natural absorption of some of the filler.

Tiny implants of a synthetic filler are sometimes used to fill skin depressions and smooth out wrinkles in the face and neck. The thread-like implants are drawn into place and anchored with a special needle. The procedure may be done without sedation using a local anesthetic. There is usually no bruising, and most patients are back to normal within a week.

Injectable fillers and synthetic implants may enhance your facial rejuvenation procedure or delay the need for surgery. Ask your facial plastic surgeon if this type of treatment is right for you.

*Occasionally, injectable fillers are used to provide a temporary improvement while a patient is considering a more permanent facial contouring procedure.*

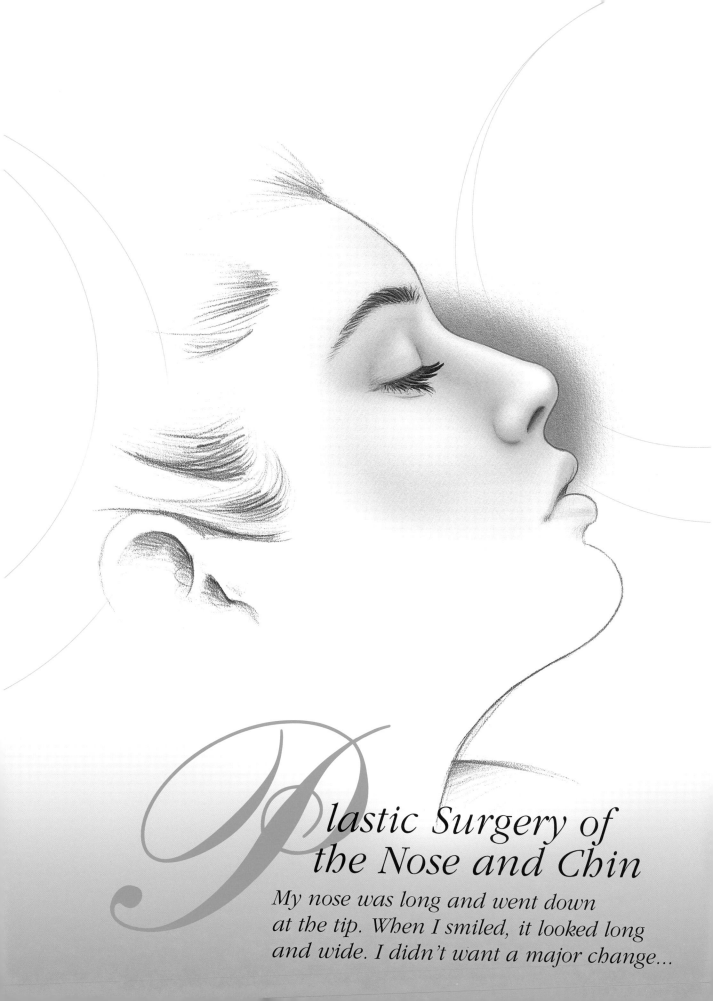

# Plastic Surgery of the Nose and Chin

*My nose was long and went down at the tip. When I smiled, it looked long and wide. I didn't want a major change...*

# Plastic Surgery of the Nose and Chin

*"My nose was long and went down at the tip. When I smiled, it looked long and wide. I didn't want a major change, and my surgery resulted in only a subtle improvement. Some people didn't even notice the change, but it made a big difference to me. It made me feel a lot better about myself."*

■ *Jennifer S., age 16*

No one feature affects the way you look quite as much as your nose. A nose that is too long, too wide, or too big can seem to dominate your face. A nose that's crooked or humped may detract from otherwise pleasing facial features. Maybe your nose has been broken. Or the tip projects too far, appears big and bulbous, or points down like a hawk's bill. Perhaps your nose just appears large because your chin is small.

Many things may be wrong with the nose you were born with. This is why more than half a million people each year consult with facial plastic surgeons about improving the shape of their nose. If your nose is not in harmony with the rest of your facial features—or if it doesn't work as well as you would like it to—you may be a candidate for nasal surgery.

Surgery to improve the appearance of the nose is called rhinoplasty. In rhinoplasty, the surgeon seeks to create a more harmonious facial appearance while maintaining or improving the breathing function of your nose. As the photographs in this chapter show, the improvement may be quite dramatic or rather subtle. Even a minor correction, however, can make a big difference in overall facial harmony.

## EVALUATING THE PROBLEM
The first step to planning a rhinoplasty procedure is a thorough examination of the nose itself—and of your reasons for wanting nasal surgery.

As Jennifer S. recalls from her initial consultation for nasal surgery, "The doctor asked why I wanted surgery, and what I didn't like about my nose. Then he looked at it and took pictures. Lots of pictures."

3
--------------
*Even a minor correction can make a big difference in overall facial harmony.*

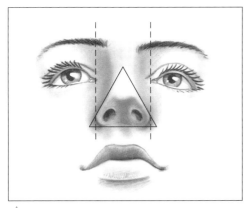

▲

*Figure 1*

*Is your nose symmetrical? Your surgeon will evaluate your nose from several different angles before surgery. From the frontal view, the nose should lie within parallel lines drawn down from the inner corners of the eyes to the nostrils. From the base view, the nasal tip should appear triangular, and the nostrils should be symmetrical in shape and size.*

A thorough screening of your attitudes and expectations is essential to planning nasal surgery. Your surgeon will want assurance that you are seeking surgery because you want it, not to please others. Also, you should demonstrate your understanding that surgery may improve your profile, not give you someone else's.

Remember, the goal of surgery is not the perfect nose, but the nose that is perfect for you. Tell your surgeon how you want your nose to look. Most people like a relatively straight nose, but a slight hump often is acceptable to men, and some women may prefer a slightly scooped shape.

In response, your surgeon will tell you if what you want is possible or suggest some alternatives, after examining your nose. Facial plastic surgeons are skilled in feeling the external nose and visualizing the cartilage and skeleton beneath. Your surgeon will examine your nose carefully, checking its symmetry and studying the strength and resilience of the cartilage and the thickness and quality of the skin. Then, your nose will be photographed and analyzed from several angles.

An important part of the evaluation includes your chin. People who want surgery to make large noses smaller are often surprised when their surgeon suggests a chin implant. This is because a weak chin can make your nose appear more prominent.

"I had never thought of it before," says Jeanine Codispotti when her surgeon suggested a chin implant. "But he was right. One of my hobbies is to draw and photograph faces, and what he said about proportion made sense to me."

▶

*Combining nasal surgery with liposhaving under the chin can transform the profile of the face.*

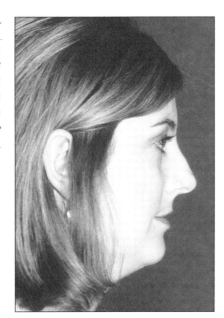
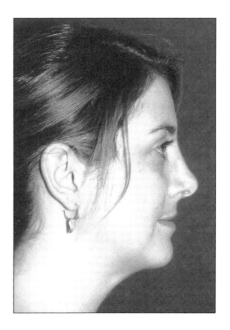

# *Picturing nasal problems*

To evaluate nasal problems, facial plastic surgeons usually photograph the nose from five different angles.

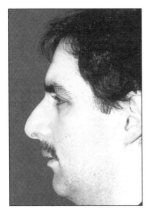

PROFILE VIEW

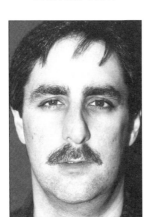

FRONTAL VIEW

A ***profile view*** shows the relationship between the brow, nose, and chin. It also allows the surgeon to measure tip projection (how far out the tip extends) and tip rotation (whether the tip is tilted up or down).

A ***frontal view*** may reveal problems with the nasal septum—the "wall" inside the nose that divides it into two chambers. Excess width and bulging in the tip also may be seen in this view. A nose should lie within lines drawn down from the inner edge of each eyebrow. Crookedness may indicate problems with the septum or other structures inside the nose.

When seen in the ***base view***, the nasal tip should appear triangular, and the nostrils should be symmetrical in shape and size. The division between the nostrils should be straight and at the midline. The width of the base should fall within parallel lines drawn straight down from the inner edge of each eye.

Halfway between the frontal and profile views is the ***oblique view***, or three-quarter view. This angle often is best for showing how the nose aligns with the cheeks and other bony and cartilaginous features.

Finally, because the nose is a dynamic feature, it may change shape when you smile. The surgeon, therefore, will evaluate the ***smiling view***, studying and photographing your face from several angles as you smile.

*Older patients seek nasal surgery for cosmetic reasons and because it helps to maintain good breathing.*

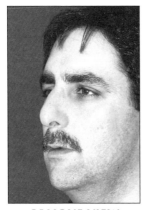

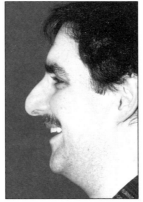

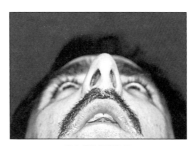

BASE VIEW

OBLIQUE VIEW                    SMILING VIEW

# *Achieving balance— the chin makes a difference*

If you feel your nose is too prominent, take a close look at your chin. It's a question of balance. A weak or receding chin line can make your nose appear bigger than it really is. A sloping forehead makes the nose seem to project even more *(see Figure 2)*.

Facial plastic surgeons are trained to look at the whole face, not just individual features. That's why patients who consult a surgeon seeking one procedure are sometimes surprised to hear the doctor suggest something different. By studying the dimensions of the face and relationships of the features to one another, the facial plastic surgeon can determine which surgical procedures are needed to create a more harmonious appearance.

To evaluate your chin, the surgeon will look at your face in profile. A vertical line drawn down from the edge of your lower lip should just touch your chin. If the tip of your chin is behind the line, chin augmentation may be needed to bring your facial features into balance. If it extends beyond the line, on the other hand, you may benefit from reduction mentoplasty, or surgery to reduce your chin size.

Chin augmentation can be done alone, or at the same time as nasal surgery. It also can accompany a facelift, liposuction of the face or neck, and other facial proce-dures. A relatively minor procedure, chin augmentation can make a big difference in the overall surgical result, even making it possible for the surgeon to do less to the nose and still achieve nice facial harmony.

The shape and projection of a small chin are improved with an implant made of special surgical plastic that mimics the feel of natural body tissues. Chin implants come in a variety of shapes and sizes, which the surgeon selects depending on the

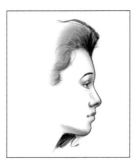 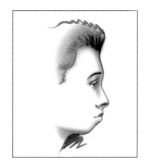 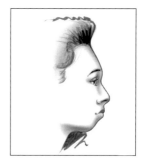

*Figure 2* ▲

*Nasal surgery or chin implant? Your nose can appear more prominent than it actually is because of other facial features. The noses in these three profiles are identical but look totally different. The face on the left, showing normal jaw structure, presents a pleasing appearance. The nose in the center profile appears more prominent because of a receding chin. And, the nose on the right seems to project even more because of a long sloping forehead and a weak chin.*

shape of the chin and the degree of correction needed. The incision is made either inside the mouth, between the lower lip and gum, or in the crease beneath the chin. The surgeon creates a small pocket and slips the implant into place. Then the incision is sutured, and a small dressing is placed on the chin.

After chin surgery, you may have a bit of swelling or feel somewhat "stretched," and you will need to avoid foods that require chewing for the first few days.

One patient recalls that her chin felt more sore than her nose, after having surgery on both features. "There was a strap around my chin, and I couldn't open my mouth very well," she notes. Within a week, however, she was able to resume her normal activities.

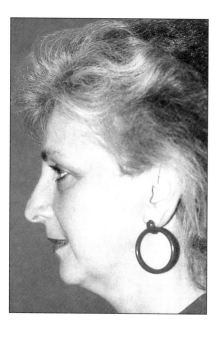 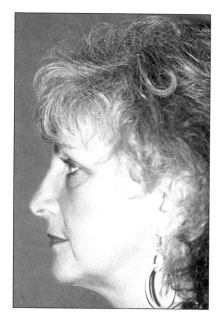

◀

*When a receding chin makes the nose seem larger than it really is, a more harmonious appearance can be achieved with rhinoplasty and chin augmentation.*

A chin that is too prominent also can be treated with a similar procedure called reduction mentoplasty. An incision is made beneath the chin, and an instrument much like a dental drill is used to shave away a small amount of excess bone.

In some cases, the chin may appear too large or too small because of a problem with the lower jaw. When this occurs, other problems, such as an overbite or seriously misaligned teeth, also may be evident. Structural problems of the jaw are corrected with a more extensive treatment known as orthognathic surgery. Because the teeth, palate, and related structures are involved, orthognathic surgery typically involves a cooperative effort involving the patient's dentist, orthodontist, and surgeon.

## THE BEST AGE FOR NASAL SURGERY

Many people wonder if there is a minimum age for nasal surgery, or if you can be too old for it.

Surgery to refine the appearance of the nose is best done after a young person has finished growing. This usually means age 13 to 15 for girls and after age 15 for boys. Sometimes, treatment is appropriate at an earlier age if an internal defect is causing serious breathing problems. In that case, however, additional surgery may be needed after the child matures. In general, it is best to wait until after puberty.

At the other end of the spectrum, nasal surgery can be done at any age as long as you are in good health. Older patients seek nasal surgery for cosmetic reasons and because it helps to maintain good breathing. As we age, nasal cartilage becomes thinner and loses its elasticity, causing the tip of the nose to lengthen and droop. Some people develop a hanging lobe between the nostrils, and the nose may appear more humped than previously. Internal breathing passages become narrower, and loose cartilage and tissue inside the nose may further obstruct the airway.

## HOW NASAL SURGERY IS DONE

Generally, the incisions needed for nose surgery are made just inside the rim of each nostril *(see Figure 3)*. Working through these incisions, the surgeon can shave away excess bone and cartilage to reduce a hump, reposition cartilage and bone to narrow the nose, and sculpt the nasal tip.

*Figure 3*
*Nasal surgery*
*incisions*

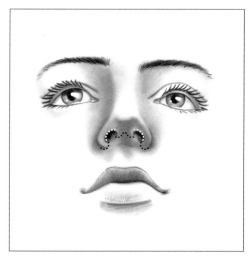

In some cases, the surgeon may make an additional incision across the base of the nose, between the nostrils. To reduce flaring nostrils, incisions also may be made on each side of the nose where the nostril joins the face. These incisions, if they are made, are usually undetectable when they heal.

Sometimes, to straighten a crooked nose or narrow its width, the nasal bone is cut. This came as a relief to one young patient.

"I thought the doctor would break my nose," she recalls, echoing a concern many patients have about nasal surgery. Instead, a fracture is made in a controlled way, so that the bones may be moved inward. It is not painful, nor does it increase bruising or swelling.

At other times, additional support is needed to strengthen drooping tissues or replace cartilage destroyed by accident or disease. In this case, the surgeon may construct a graft or strut from your own cartilage and stitch it into place. This technique may be used to increase tip projection or correct a depression in the bridge of the nose.

After correcting the framework of the nose, the skin is redraped and the incisions are closed with absorbable sutures. A small splint may be applied to the outside of your nose to support it while it heals, and absorbent dressing material may be placed inside.

Nasal surgery may be done under light intravenous sedation with local anesthesia, often in an ambulatory care center or an operating facility located right in the surgeon's office. General anesthesia is preferred in some cases—if the surgery is very extensive, for instance, or if you are especially nervous. In that case you may spend a night in the hospital.

## IMPROVING THE FUNCTION OF THE NOSE

If your initial evaluation reveals obstructions in your nose that are causing difficult breathing, chronic sinus problems, or recurring headaches, a procedure called septorhinoplasty may be performed.

This procedure can improve both the function and appearance of your nose. Through incisions placed inside the nostrils, the surgeon straightens the nasal septum—the wall that divides the nose into two chambers—and removes any excess tissue that interferes with air flow.

Jeanine Codispotti recently learned she was an ideal candidate for a septorhinoplasty. After breaking her nose during her teens, she developed a nasal hump and a deviated septum.

"My nice, straight nose grew larger, too, and didn't look right to me," she says, "and I began to have trouble breathing."

For years, Jeanine took sinus medicine, but eventually developed a severe reaction to the medication. "That was when I decided to look into nasal surgery," she says. Her surgeon removed the hump and straightened her nasal septum. He also suggested a chin implant, to improve the overall harmony of her face. "I can breathe freely without medication now," she says happily, "and my nose is just the way I remember it. I really like the way I look now!"

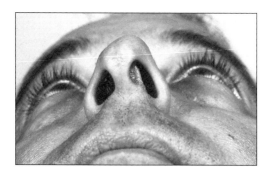 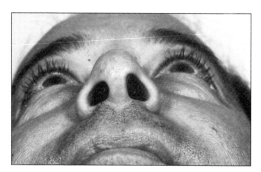

*Asymmetrical noses often indicate breathing problems, which septorhinoplasty can correct.*

## AFTER THE SURGERY

Most patients report little or no pain after nasal surgery, and any discomfort is easily controlled with mild pain medication. Your nose will be stuffy for a few days, but you must not blow your nose for at least a week. Your surgeon may give you an oral decongestant to make you more comfortable. If you wear glasses, they must not put pressure on your nose for the first two weeks. Your surgeon will advise you on how to keep the weight of your glasses off your nose by using tape or a support device.

Internal nasal dressing, if it is used, generally is removed the day after surgery. The splint remains on for five to eight days. You should expect to experience some swelling and bruising around your eyes. Cold compresses will help reduce this and make you feel more comfortable. Most of the swelling subsides in about three weeks, and any remaining bruises can be covered with makeup about a week after surgery.

Don't be too surprised if you experience a bit of emotional turmoil immediately after surgery. "After the procedure, I felt a little down," Jeanine explains. "I thought about my nose constantly and kept questioning whether I had done the right thing. Once the packing was taken out, I felt better and my spirits lifted."

A nice thing about nasal surgery is that your nose continues to improve for several months. It takes at least six months for most of the swelling to subside. Deeper healing of the nasal tissues takes even longer, and subtle refinements may still occur a year or more after surgery.

*Here, a minor change narrows the nose, giving the face greater definition.*

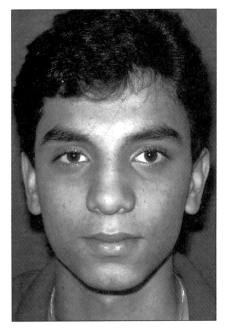 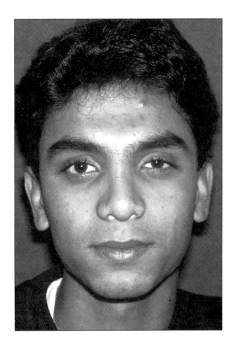

# *Revision rhinoplasty— correcting serious problems*

Julie Kern was only 15 when she had nasal surgery with disappointing results. "It looked awful," Julie says. "My nose looked flattened and the tip was too small. Even worse, I developed breathing problems."

Twice during the years that followed, Julie had surgery to repair her nose, without success. The years that followed were torture for Julie. "Every day I had to look at it in the mirror and I just wanted to cry," she reports. "I had been doing some modeling at the time and I had to give it up. I developed an anxiety disorder. A day never went by without someone asking me, 'What happened to your nose?' It affected my whole life."

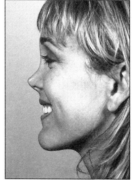

Julie went to one doctor after another, searching for answers. "I contacted doctors in other states and even in Europe," she says. "Some said they could fix it, but I didn't trust anyone anymore."

*Remember, the goal of surgery is not the perfect nose, but the nose that is perfect for you.*

Julie didn't give up, however, and she finally found the facial plastic surgeon who changed her life. "I knew right away he was different," she says. "He had a lot of pictures, showing how he had repaired other noses like mine. The pictures gave me confidence." Even so, it took nearly a year for Julie to build up enough nerve to go through with the surgery.

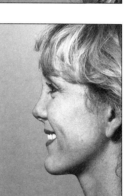

The surgeon used a synthetic material to create a new nasal bridge for Julie. Because so much of her nasal cartilage had been removed, he took cartilage from her ears to reconstruct the septum and nasal tip. Julie is ecstatic with the results. "It looked better right away," she said. "There was hardly any bruising, and I went out to dinner just a week after the surgery."

Although Julie's experience is an unusual one, it demonstrates how facial plastic surgeons can use special techniques to repair damaged noses. Surgery intended to correct problems that appear after an earlier procedure is called revision rhinoplasty. Because it is more complex than an initial procedure, it should not be taken lightly. When serious problems exist, however, revision rhinoplasty may offer hope. Similar techniques also are used to restore form and function to a nose damaged by serious illness or traumatic injury.

The revision procedure changed Julie's life. "I have confidence now that I never had before," she says. "Before, my nose was the first thing anyone noticed about me. Now, no one can tell there was ever anything wrong."

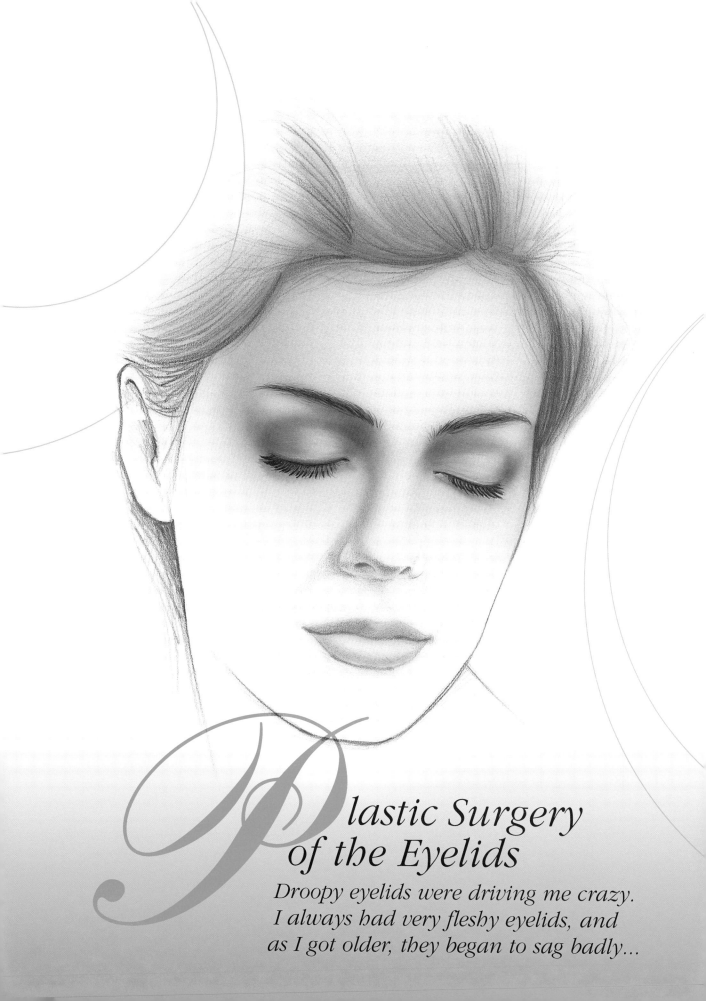

# Plastic Surgery of the Eyelids

*Droopy eyelids were driving me crazy.*
*I always had very fleshy eyelids, and*
*as I got older, they began to sag badly...*

# Plastic Surgery of the Eyelids

*"Droopy eyelids were driving me crazy. I had always had very fleshy eyelids, and as I got older, they began to sag badly. Putting on makeup was difficult. My eyelids felt funny, too, like they were in my way. Without realizing it, I started keeping my brow muscles tensed upward all the time. I was shocked when I saw that I had developed permanent creases in my forehead from doing that."*

■ *Agnes W., age 58*

When it comes to expressing your deepest thoughts and emotions, there is probably no facial feature quite as important as your eyes. When they look tired, saggy, or puffy, more than just your appearance may suffer—the image you project to others is affected as well.

"People were always saying I looked tired," comments Stephanie Chism, age 33. "My eyes seemed puffy all the time, so it's not surprising, but I didn't like hearing it—especially when I felt just fine."

Drooping, overhung upper lids and sagging lower lids can happen to anyone. Eyelid problems often are one of the first signs of aging, but even young people can be affected. Chronic allergies can cause the eyelids to swell, speeding the development of overhanging upper lids or bags under the eyes. Sun exposure, excess squinting, and habitual eye-rubbing can promote sagginess. Heredity also plays a part.

"My dad had heavy brows and lids like mine," Stephanie notes. "I decided to get something done while I was still young, because I could see that the problem would only get worse."

4

*If your eyes make you seem droopy, sad, or tired, blepharoplasty can open them up dramatically and give you a fresher, brighter, more youthful appearance.*

Fortunately, eyelid problems can be treated very effectively through blepharoplasty, a relatively simple procedure that removes excess skin, muscle, and fatty tissue. It often is combined with other facial plastic surgery procedures, such as browlift, facelift, or skin resurfacing.

If your eyes make you seem droopy, sad, or tired, blepharoplasty can open them up dramatically and give you a fresher, brighter, more youthful appearance.

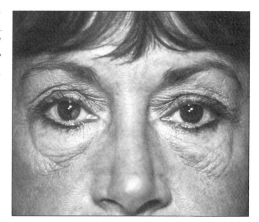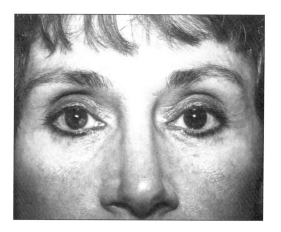

*Blepharoplasty can rejuvenate an aging face.*

## WHY EYELIDS SAG

Everyone experiences changes in the eyelids over time. Every time you blink—and you blink billions of times over the course of your lifetime—the skin and muscles of your upper eyelids stretch a bit. Elastic fibers in the skin draw them back to their natural position. Imagine what happens to a rubber band when you stretch it out and snap it back repeatedly, and you can easily see what happens in your eyelid—over time, the skin and muscles of the upper eyelid get longer.

Eventually, a little fold of skin may develop as the excess skin bulges outward and hangs over the lid. In some people, the overhanging skin actually rests on the eyelashes, causing an uncomfortable sensation and making it difficult to look upward. You may notice your

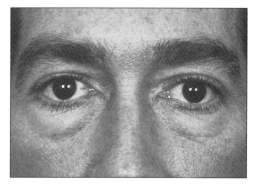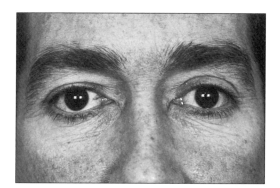

*A more refreshed look is often the result when under-eye bags are improved with blepharoplasty.*

eyelids sticking momentarily when you blink, and, if you are a woman, you may find it diffi-cult to apply eye makeup. If the problem is severe enough, you may even find your vision obscured by the drooping upper lids. In this case, your insurance plan may cover a portion of the cost of treatment.

Sagging in the lower lids is sometimes described as having "bags under the eyes." Nearly everyone develops some degree of sagging in this area. Gravity and age are the biggest culprits, but even young people may have excess fat deposits under the eyes.

"It was a family trait," says Connie H., age 46. "I have always had bags under my eyes. I hated to look in the mirror. Now that I've had them done, everyone says I look great, but no one can put their finger on what the difference is."

The eyes are surrounded by a protective layer of fatty tissue encased in a membrane that holds it tightly in place. Over time, the membrane can weaken, allowing the fatty tissue to slip downward. Skin and muscle are stretched by the protruding tissue, producing puffy bulges that are impossible to hide with cosmetics.

The problem often is worst in the morning, because fluid collects in the fatty tissue while you are lying down. Gravity may draw the fluid away after you get up in the morning, but if you have a great deal of excess fatty tissue, it may take a long time to clear up.

*In some people, the overhanging skin actually rests on the eyelashes, causing an uncomfortable sensation and making it difficult to look upward.*

Blepharoplasty removes excess skin in the upper and lower lids and reduces the amount of fatty tissue under the eye. Surgery may be done on the upper or the lower lids, or both, depending on the specific problem.

## HOW BLEPHAROPLASTY IS DONE

Incisions in the upper lids are made in the crease above each eye *(see Figure 1)*. Excess muscle, fat, and loose skin are removed, and fine sutures are used to close the incisions. The resulting scar normally fades to a fine line that virtually disappears into the eyelid crease.

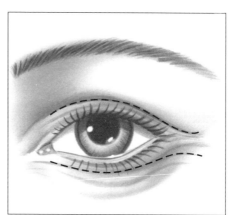

*Figure 1*
*External incisions*

To remove excess fatty tissue below the eye, inci-sions may be made just inside the lower eyelid, on the pink part that you see when you pull your eyelid downward *(see Figure 2)*. This is called a transconjunctival approach. The incisions may be closed with tiny sutures that dissolve within a few days, or they may not be sutured at all. If excess skin or muscle needs to be removed, the incision may be made in a natural smile crease below the lashline *(see Figure 1)*.

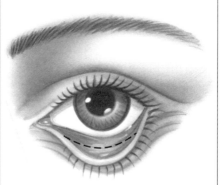

*Figure 2*
*Transconjunctival incision*

Eyelid surgery usually is performed under intravenous sedation and local anesthesia, often in an ambulatory surgical center or an office surgery facility. Most people go home the same day.

"I was aware of the surgery, but I was totally relaxed and kept drifting in and out" is the way one patient describes the surgery. "I don't remember a thing," maintains another.

You may experience some mild swelling or bruising of your eyelids after surgery, but this usually subsides quickly. Your surgeon may recommend using cold compresses and keeping your head elevated when you lie down to help reduce swelling and speed healing. If you have any discomfort after surgery, it can be controlled with mild pain medications.

"I felt some discomfort, but no real pain," says Connie H. "Although I took two weeks off, I was called in to work a shift just a few days after surgery, and I did fine, stitches and all."

Eyelids heal remarkably quickly and scars usually are quite inconspicuous. Women can completely camouflage any remaining marks with eye makeup. Most men find that the scars disappear into their natural "smile" lines. Most people return to their normal routine within a week after surgery. It may help to wear dark glasses for a few days, both to cover the swelling and to remind you not to touch your eyelids while they heal. If you wear contact lenses, you must wait two to three weeks before you can resume wearing them.

"The first couple of days were the hardest," Agnes W. recalls. "By the fifth day, I was just glad I did it. The bruising lasted several weeks, but I concealed it with makeup. The procedure made a dramatic difference in the way I look, and I was surprised at how much better it made me feel."

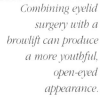

*Combining eyelid surgery with a browlift can produce a more youthful, open-eyed appearance.*

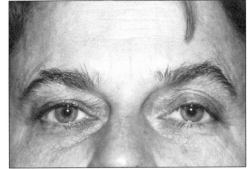 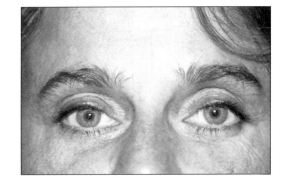

# *Surgery to modify Asian eyes*

People of Asian descent sometimes request eye surgery designed to create a double eyelid. Typically, the Asian eyelid hangs like a smooth curtain from the brow to the lashes. The double eyelid procedure creates a fold that separates the eyelid into two portions.

Blepharoplasty to create a double eyelid is often done during the teen years. It is most often sought by young women of Asian descent, but it also is appropriate for older patients and men.

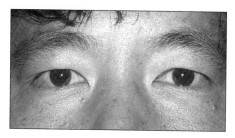 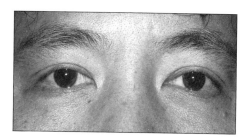

*Eyelids heal remarkably quickly and scars are usually quite inconspicuous.*

Although the desire for a double eyelid is common among some people of Asian heritage, it does not necessarily indicate a preference for a "Western" appearance. Many patients requesting surgery simply want a more "open-eyed" look. Some have heavy eyelids that interfere with their vision. Others have an unusually narrow eye opening that causes problems when wearing contact lenses or applying cosmetics.

To create a double eyelid, the surgeon makes an incision in the upper lid above the lash line, removes a small amount of fatty tissue, and places sutures in the lid and muscle to create a fold. The procedure can be done in a way that provides a subtle enhancement while preserving a distinctive Asian appearance.

Surgery is performed with local anesthesia and mild intravenous sedation that allow you to be relaxed but awake. This is because you will need to open your eyes during the procedure so the surgeon can check for symmetry and determine that the eyelid will function properly.

Some swelling and bruising may follow surgery, but most of it subsides quickly. Scars are well hidden in the newly created fold of the double eyelid, and most patients can return to a normal routine within seven to 10 days after the procedure.

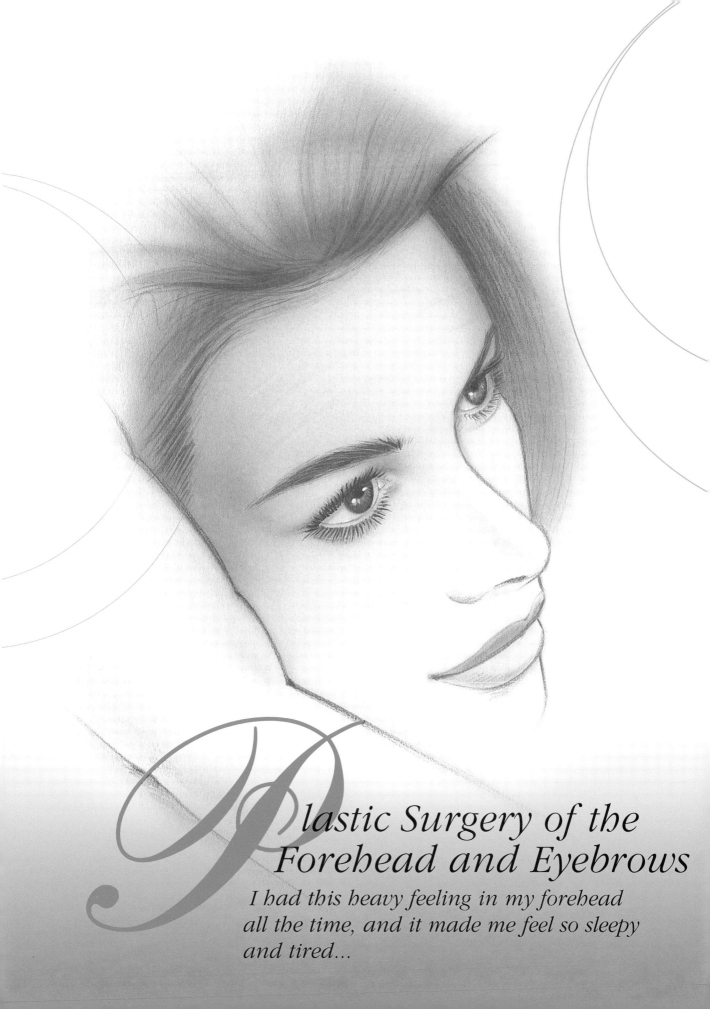

# Plastic Surgery of the Forehead and Eyebrows

*I had this heavy feeling in my forehead
all the time, and it made me feel so sleepy
and tired...*

# Plastic Surgery of the Forehead and Eyebrows

*"I had this heavy feeling in my forehead all the time, and it made me feel so sleepy and tired. Sometimes I would grab my forehead and pull up, just for a moment's relief. Then I noticed that I was losing my peripheral vision—my drooping eyebrows actually were in the way. I went to a facial plastic surgeon, and after a direct browlift and an eyelid tuck, it's like a big weight has been taken off my head. The surgery was not difficult, and now I feel refreshed. It's a good feeling."*

■ *Doug Gast, age 51*

If stress, time, and the elements have conspired to give you a permanently worried look, you're not alone. A wrinkled forehead and sagging eyebrows are early signs of aging in many people, and the problem generally gets worse as time goes on. Heredity can also play a role, because heavy eyebrows run in families. When brows overshadow the eyes, even young people can look prematurely tired.

"People always thought I looked severe, even grumpy," says Marta B., who finally had a browlift at age 51. "By then, everything had fallen—including my eyebrows, which sagged below the underlying bone." Marta's surgery transformed what she felt was a perpetually haggard expression into a more alert, youthful look. In her words, "It took years off my appearance."

As Marta learned, the eyebrows are an important feature of the upper face, particularly for conveying emotions. They frame the eyes, define the brow, and enhance the expression of

5

---

*High, arched eyebrows convey a youthful appearance. Droopy brows can make you look older and sadder than you feel.*

the eyes. High, arched eyebrows convey a youthful appearance. Droopy brows, on the other hand, can make you look older and sadder than you feel. Likewise, frown lines or permanent creases between the eyebrows can make even the calmest person appear tense or angry.

Browlift is the general term used to refer to a variety of surgical techniques designed to correct sagging in the forehead area. Browlift procedures can raise and reshape the eyebrows, lift and tighten the forehead skin, and relax vertical creases between the eyebrows. Not uncommonly, they are done in conjunction with other facial plastic surgery procedures—such as an eyelid tuck, facelift, or skin resurfacing—as part of a coordinated facial rejuvenation plan.

## CHOOSING THE BEST TECHNIQUE

The browlift technique your surgeon chooses will depend on the nature and severity of your problem, the degree of correction desired, your age, the elasticity of your skin, and whether you are a man or a woman.

In selecting the technique most appropriate for you, the surgeon will want you to explain exactly what you believe the problem to be and what you hope the surgery will accomplish.

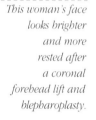

*This woman's face looks brighter and more rested after a coronal forehead lift and blepharoplasty.*

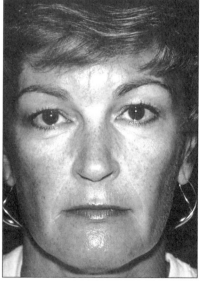 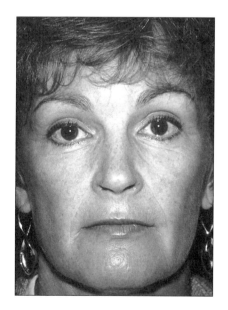

Don't be surprised if the doctor asks how you normally wear your hair or how you feel about the creases in your forehead. The answers to questions like these will help determine which technique to use and the placement of incisions.

"I really wasn't worried about wrinkles and creases," recalls Doug Gast. "I just wanted to regain my peripheral vision and end that constant sensation of heaviness, like my brows were overhanging my eyes."

Doug was helped with a procedure called an indirect eyebrow lift. "The surgeon chose two forehead crease lines, one on each side of my forehead, and made the incisions there," he explains. "The scars are hidden by the creases and are barely noticeable" *(see Figure 1)*.

Because the indirect eyebrow lift relies on natural creases to hide the scars, it is often more acceptable to men. Women, on the other hand, may benefit from a coronal lift, which lifts and smoothes the entire forehead area. The incision for a coronal lift usually is made just behind the natural hairline, across the top of the head *(see Figure 2)*.

Connie H., a hairdresser, had a coronal lift at age 46. "The procedure smoothed out the wrinkles in my forehead and restored a nice, natural arch to my eyebrows," she says.

The coronal lift generally is not suitable for men who may later experience male pattern baldness because it may elevate the hairline somewhat. In women with high hairlines, the incision can be placed just within the hairline. The incision is made on an angle, which allows the hair to grow through the scar, effectively camouflaging it *(see Figure 2)*. Since no hair-bearing skin is removed, this procedure—called a high forehead lift—can actually lower the hairline a bit.

A direct eyebrow lift may be recommended for men who are likely to have hair loss, as well as for women who do not have loose skin or wrinkling in the forehead area. The incisions for a direct eyebrow lift are made just within or above each eyebrow *(see Figure 1)*. The scar normally fades to a narrow line that may be camouflaged with makeup, if desired.

A midforehead lift often is appropriate for men who have an abundance of forehead creases. A modification of the coronal lift, the technique involves a single incision made directly across the forehead, using natural creases to camouflage the scar *(see Figure 1)*. Unlike the coronal lift, the midforehead lift does not elevate the hairline. It allows more tightening of the skin and muscles than a direct eyebrow lift and enables the surgeon to tighten loose skin between the eyebrows as well as on the sides.

Endoscopic browlift is a less invasive technique for elevating the eyebrows and smoothing out worry lines. It is done by inserting a tiny viewing device called an endoscope and specialized surgical instruments through several half-inch incisions made within or just behind the hairline *(see Figure 2)*. This procedure repositions excess forehead skin, rather

*Because the indirect eyebrow lift relies on natural creases to hide the scars, it is often more acceptable to men. Women may benefit from a coronal lift, which lifts and smoothes the entire forehead area.*

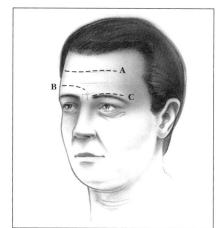

◄

*Figure 1*

A. *Midforehead lift incision*
B. *Indirect browlift incision*
C. *Direct browlift incision*

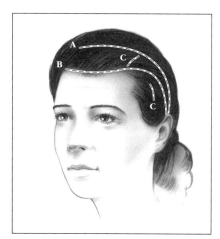

◄

*Figure 2*

A. *Coronal lift incision*
B. *High forehead lift incision*
C. *Endoscopic browlift incisions*

than removing it. Your facial plastic surgeon will determine if it is an appropriate technique for your needs.

## HOW THE PROCEDURE IS DONE

*Endoscopic surgery of the forehead includes a wide range of options, from a relatively simple technique for fixing sagging eyebrows in place to more complex procedures for lifting and smoothing the entire forehead area.*

Browlift surgery generally is done in an ambulatory surgical center or an office surgery facility. Intravenous sedation and local anesthesia are used to keep you comfortable during the procedure. Most people go home the same day.

In a coronal, high forehead, or midforehead lift, the forehead and eyebrows are elevated, excess skin is removed, and sutures or surgical staples are used to close the incision. This type of lift repositions the eyebrows, smoothes out horizontal creases, and diminishes wrinkles between the eyes.

In a direct or indirect eyebrow lift, the surgeon removes a small wedge of excess skin above each eyebrow and places permanent sutures in the underlying muscles to hold them in their new position. An eyebrow lift improves the position and appearance of the eyebrows, but has little effect on forehead creases or worry lines between the eyes.

Endoscopic surgery of the forehead includes a wide range of options, from a relatively simple technique for fixing sagging eyebrows in place to more complex procedures for lifting and smoothing the entire forehead area. Working with special instruments inserted through small incisions, the surgeon lifts and tightens muscles, fixing them in place with permanent sutures or tiny screws.

After the surgery, your incisions may be covered with a light dressing, or they may be left uncovered. You may be given a tight headband to wear for several days to hold your eyebrows in place while the area heals.

*A browlift and blepharoplasty can be performed at the same time as a facelift and skin resurfacing for optimum results.*

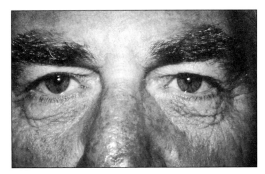 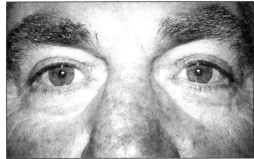

You should expect some swelling or bruising during the first 10 days after surgery, but this can be kept to a minimum by keeping your head elevated—especially at night—and using cold compresses. You also may notice some numbness in your scalp. This almost always diminishes over time as healing progresses.

# "I'm so glad I did this!"

Browlift surgery can be part of a more extensive procedure, as Ruth Yag, who is 61, learned when she consulted a facial plastic surgeon about a droopy eyebrow.

"My left eyebrow always had a tendency to droop slightly," she explains. "It started getting worse a few years ago, and soon I could look up and see my eyebrow hanging down and pressing against my eyelid."

Ruth thought an eyelid lift might solve her problem, until her surgeon pointed out the laxness in the muscles supporting her brow. Ruth accepted her surgeon's suggestion and opted for a coronal lift, an upper eyelid tuck, and a medium chemical peel under her eyes.

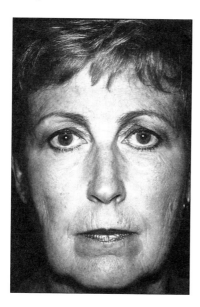 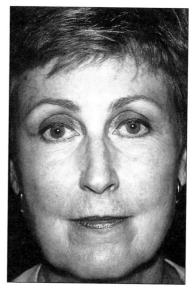

The procedures were done in the doctor's office surgery facility under twilight anesthesia. The entire process took about three hours, but Ruth was not aware of the details. "I went into the operating room, and the next thing I remember is sitting in my recliner at home with my husband. I don't even remember how I got there."

Afterwards, she says, there was very little swelling or bruising and hardly any pain. "I expected it to be quite painful, but truthfully, it wasn't. I didn't even need the medication he prescribed. The staples in the long hairline incision pulled and itched a little as the skin healed, but I did exactly as he told me—using ice and keeping it elevated—and the incision healed quickly."

In two weeks, Ruth was ready to resume her normal activities. "The droop was gone and my eyes were more open. The best part was that I could see better. That was a nice surprise."

Her facial plastic surgery experience was an unqualified success, Ruth concludes. "I am so glad I did this. I would recommend it to anyone."

Most patients resume a normal routine about two weeks after surgery, although you will be advised to avoid strenuous physical activity for approximately six weeks. Sutures usually are removed seven to 10 days following surgery, and makeup may be applied to camouflage any remaining scars.

"I honestly had no pain," says Marta B., whose browlift was performed endoscopically. "There was some discomfort, but it was just a mild annoyance. I had a lot of swelling for the first five days and the top of my head felt numb and tight. I had some bruising under one of my eyes, too, but all that went away quickly. I attended a party two weeks after my surgery, and no one suspected a thing. I got a lot of compliments, though, on how great I looked."

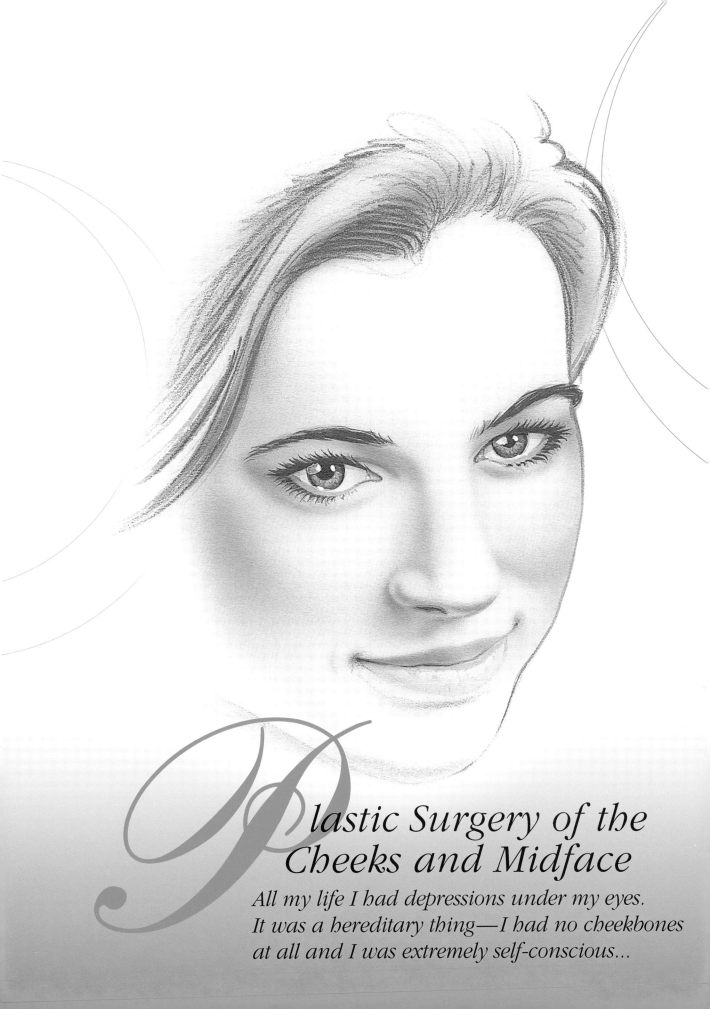

# Plastic Surgery of the Cheeks and Midface

*All my life I had depressions under my eyes.
It was a hereditary thing—I had no cheekbones
at all and I was extremely self-conscious...*

# Plastic Surgery of the Cheeks and Midface

*"All my life I had depressions under my eyes. It was a hereditary thing—I had no cheekbones at all and I was extremely self-conscious about it. Although I didn't need glasses, I wore them to camouflage the problem. It might seem like a small thing, but it was hard for me to deal with. I'm thrilled with the way cheek implants made me look. I am so much more confident now."*

■ *Laurie Griffith, age 33*

There's no doubt about it: Good cheekbones are an important part of good looks. Cheekbones help define the face. They highlight the eyes, add balance to the facial features, and contribute to an appearance of youth and vigor.

Not everyone is born with good cheekbones. If yours are underdeveloped, you may feel that your face looks somewhat flat and expressionless. The problem may become more apparent as you age and your cheeks take on a more hollow appearance.

Suzanne A. can relate to this: "I never really had much in the way of cheekbones," she relates. "After 40, my cheeks began to have a more sunken appearance. Friends were always saying I looked tired, even though I wasn't."

The solution for Suzanne was a procedure known as malar augmentation, or, to put it simply, cheek implants.

"The procedure raised everything up and gave me a fresher, more refined look," Suzanne says. "It was a very subtle difference—in fact, nobody knew I had anything done. But to me, it helped a lot."

6

*Cheekbones help define the face. They highlight the eyes, add balance to the facial features, and contribute to an appearance of youth and vigor.*

*The contour
of your
midface region
involves more
than just your
cheekbones.*

Cheek implants often are done in conjunction with other procedures. Because they enhance facial harmony, they sometimes are recommended to patients seeking to reduce the prominence of a nose or chin. More often, they are done along with facial rejuvenation procedures.

"My first concern was the bags under my eyes," recalls Marilyn A., who sought the advice of a facial plastic surgeon at age 43. "As I thought about it, I realized that attractive people tend to have nice cheekbones—and I simply didn't. I discussed it with the surgeon, who agreed that an implant to fill out my cheeks and midface would give me nicer definition and a more youthful appearance."

Marilyn went ahead with a combined procedure that included a midfacial implant, lower lid blepharoplasty, and a mild chemical peel. "I no longer have that drawn look," she says now. "I feel pretty again."

## EVALUATING YOUR MIDFACE REGION

The contour of your midface region involves more than just your cheekbones. The soft tissues of the midface region and the fat pad of the cheeks also come into play, as well as the structure of your jaw, chin, nose and other features. For this reason, your surgeon will analyze your entire face carefully, taking all your features into account. Small cheekbones, for example, may make your nose appear more prominent than it is, and a large, square jaw line may overpower the upper part of your face. The surgeon also will evaluate the texture of your skin, the quality and thickness of the fat under the skin, and the contours of your underlying bone structure to determine the best placement of a midfacial implant.

Augmentation of the midface region no longer means simply placing an implant over the cheekbone to build it up. Several types of implants, made of a surgical-grade synthetic

▶

*Cheek augmentation
and blepharoplasty
have given
this patient a more
youthful, less drawn
appearance.*

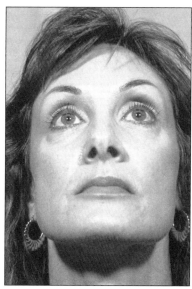
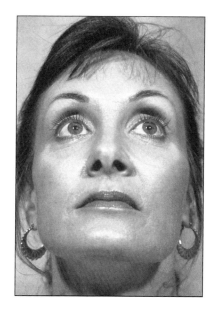

material, are available in different sizes to improve the bone structure, correct specific problems, and augment the soft tissues of the midface. The newer implants, which were designed by means of advanced, three-dimensional computer technology, allow facial plastic surgeons to achieve a more natural result in contouring the midfacial region.

The fat pad of the cheek and other soft tissues tend to slip down with age, causing hollow depressions to appear below the cheeks and deep folds to develop around the mouth. This can happen to anyone, although the problem is particularly noticeable if the underlying bone structure is inadequate. Modern facial augmentation procedures not only create natural-looking, attractive cheekbones, but they also can restore a more youthful contour to the midfacial area.

This was the experience of Mary C., who had implants placed in her cheeks and chin at the same time. "My face—which was always long and thin—had narrowed with age, making me look haggard and drawn," she explains. "When I asked about a facelift, the surgeon explained that my face needed more structure to hold the soft tissue in place."

The solution for Mary was submalar augmentation—implants placed below the cheekbones to support the sagging soft tissues of the midface. "The implants subtly round out my face and give me a softer look. The chin implant smoothed out the line of my jaw and added balance. It was such a simple procedure, but the results were unbelievable. No one believes I'm 51."

As Mary learned, submalar implants often are done before a facelift is needed, to restore youthful vitality to a face that has begun to have a sunken appearance. The procedure also may be done in conjunction with a facelift, to provide needed support for the lifted tissues.

## PLACING THE IMPLANTS

Cheek implants normally are inserted through incisions made inside the mouth, between the upper gums and the cheek. The surgeon creates a pocket over the cheekbone and slides the implant into place, closing the incisions with sutures that dissolve over time.

The procedure usually is performed under mild intravenous sedation and local anesthesia. It typically is done in an ambulatory surgical center or an office surgery facility.

"I don't remember anything about the surgery," says Mary. "The whole process was very comfortable."

After the procedure, you should follow your surgeon's instructions carefully to promote rapid healing. You may be advised not to brush your teeth until the incisions heal, and you will have to eat only liquids or very soft foods for several days. Some doctors may have you wear a pressure bandage for several days to keep the implants firmly in place.

"I looked like a bank robber," laughs Marilyn. "I stayed in for two days, and kept ice on my face to reduce swelling."

*The fat pad of the cheek and other soft tissues tend to slip down with age, causing hollow depressions to appear below the cheeks and deep folds to develop around the mouth.*

*The newer implants, which were designed by means of advanced, three-dimensional computer technology, allow facial plastic surgeons to achieve a more natural result in contouring the midfacial region.*

Most people return to work within a week after a facial implant procedure. Expect some swelling at first, but it will diminish within two weeks or so. You should see your new facial contours emerging within four to six weeks. Supportive tissue forms around the implant as it heals, and after a few weeks, you won't be able to tell the implant from your normal bone structure.

"I'm so happy I did this," Suzanne concludes. "It looks so natural, and I love what it's done for my face—and my spirits! I feel young and attractive again."

▶

*Several types of implants are used to augment the soft tissues of the midface.*

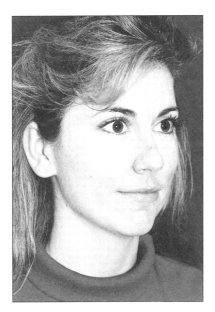 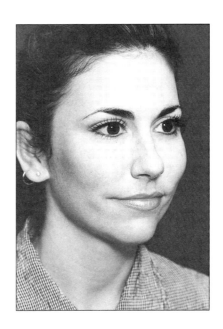

# *Techniques for enhancing the lips*

Just as soft, round, firm cheeks convey an aura of youth and good health, so do well-defined, shapely lips. Unfortunately, lips—like cheeks—are subject to sagging as we age. The problem is especially noticeable in women who were endowed by nature with thin lips. Even those born with "perfect" lips, however, will find that as time goes on, the colored portion of the lips thins out, and the arch of the upper lip—called "Cupid's bow"—flattens.

Several facial plastic surgery techniques are available to enhance the fullness of lips and create and maintain a pleasing lip contour. One option is to augment the lip line with injections of purified collagen, a protein derived from cows. Collagen plumps up the border of the lips and raises the droopy corners, but it may not last more than a few months. Fat taken from elsewhere in your body can be injected into the lips to provide volume. The fat usually is reabsorbed after about a month, although some doctors report that subsequent treatments produce more long-lasting results.

Surgical lip advancement offers a more permanent solution for some people. In this relatively simple procedure, an incision is made along the line where the colored part of the lip meets the skin—what surgeons call the vermilion border. A tiny strip of white skin is removed and the red lip edge is advanced outward and stitched in place. The incisions heal quickly and scars are usually imperceptible. The procedure usually provides the most satisfactory results to patients who have experienced thinning of the lips due to age.

If you have naturally thin lips, you may benefit from a lip implant procedure. Thin strips of an inert surgical synthetic material are threaded into the lips by means of a special needle. The implant adds bulk to naturally thin lips and restores fullness to lips that have thinned as a result of age. The implant can be placed without sedation using a local anesthetic. There is usually no bruising, and most patients find that they are back to normal within a week. Because the implant material lasts indefinitely, the shape and fullness of your lips are enhanced permanently.

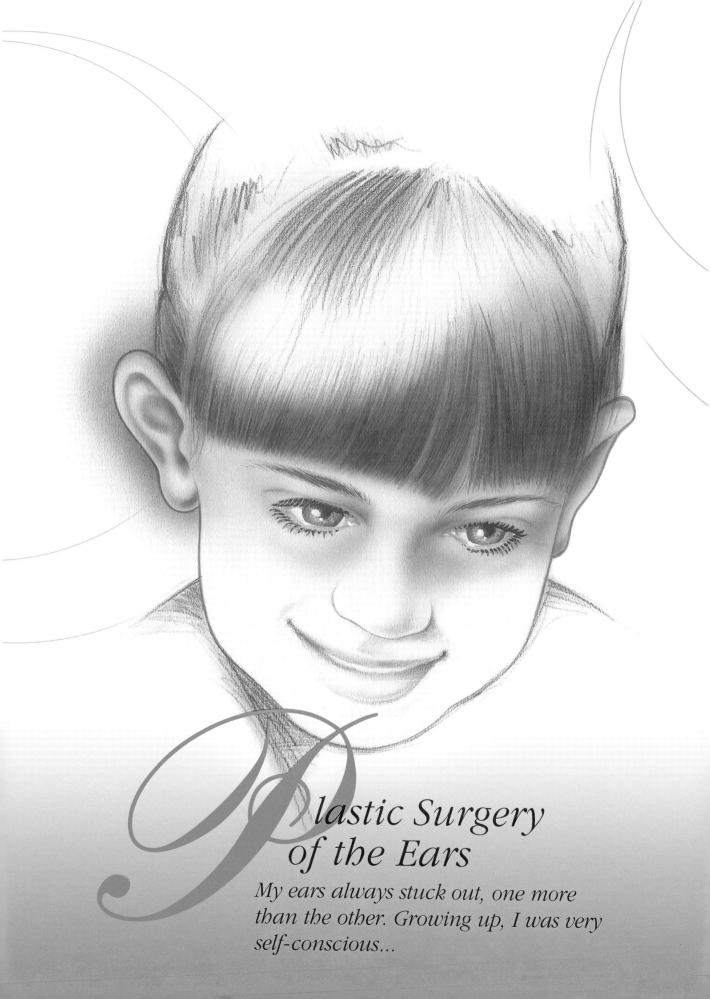

# Plastic Surgery of the Ears

*My ears always stuck out, one more than the other. Growing up, I was very self-conscious...*

# Plastic Surgery of the Ears

*"My ears always stuck out, one more than the other. Growing up, I was very self-conscious. I never wore my hair in a pony tail. It was awful when I went swimming because when my hair got wet, my ears would stick through it. I hated the way they looked. Now that I've had surgery, I definitely feel better about my appearance."*

■ *Joanne J., age 43*

Do your ears stick out too much? Are they too large, misshapen, or uneven? You may not think of ears as a particularly important beauty attribute, but they do have an impact on overall appearance. Ears that are out of proportion with the rest of the face can attract unkind remarks.

"I don't think people realize how protruding ears can affect a child growing up," says Traci B., who had ear surgery at the age of 22. "As a youngster, my ears—and the fact that I was tall and thin—made me incredibly conscious of my appearance. I styled my hair to hide my ears, and I was always careful never to do anything that might call attention to them. I avoided sports, which I love, because I wouldn't tie my hair back."

Covering his ears with long hair was not an option for Todd B., who suffered the inevitable teasing until he finally had surgery in his senior year of high school.

"It bothered me, but I learned to deal with it," Todd recalls.

Although most children with physical flaws do survive childhood teasing and grow into well-adjusted adulthood, few look back and say they are glad it happened. Nor does it have to. Ear abnormalities may be improved relatively easily through a facial plastic surgery procedure called otoplasty.

7

*"I styled my hair to hide my ears, and I was always careful never to do anything that might call attention to them. I avoided sports, which I love, because I wouldn't tie my hair back."*

## ABOUT EAR ABNORMALITIES

Ear problems tend to run in families. In those families, for reasons no one fully understands, the development of the outer ears stops short in the womb. Normally, the ears begin to take shape early in pregnancy. Delicate structures of cartilage and soft tissue covered by a thin layer of skin, the ears first stick straight out. Then, as the natural folds of the ear develop, they gradually assume a position closer to the head. By the time of birth, a baby's outer ears have achieved the complex arrangement of folds that give the ear its characteristic shape.

When prenatal development is curtailed, the normal folds may fail to develop, and the child is born with cuplike ears that project from the side of the head. In other cases, excess ear cartilage develops, resulting in normally shaped ears that stick out too far. Occasionally, the ears just grow to be too large. Because each ear develops independently, it is not uncommon for one ear to protrude more than the other, or have a noticeably different shape, giving the person an unbalanced look.

As we age, the outer ear undergoes more changes. Collagen fibers relax with time, and the ears of older people develop telltale creases and elongated earlobes.

# *The ideal ear*

Nice ears may take almost any shape. The way they affect your appearance is determined primarily by the way they harmonize your face and head. Most people prefer ears that lie close to the head and extend from the level of the brow to the base of the nose *(see Figure 1)*. Ears that are out of proportion with the rest of the face can draw too much attention to themselves, marring the appearance of even the most attractive person.

Earlobes usually take one of two shapes: straight and attached at the side of the head, or curved and hanging. With age, earlobes grow, becoming longer at the base. Earlobe problems—such as excessively long, asymmetrical, or overly blunt lobes—also may be treated through ear surgery.

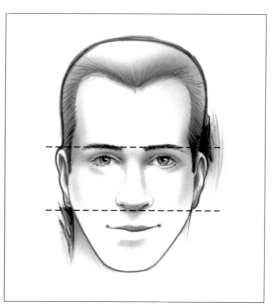

*Figure 1*

Otoplasty can help improve abnormally shaped ears, young or old. Interestingly, a change in shape will not affect hearing. Although the ears' folds and convolutions do serve to concentrate and localize sound waves, routine surgery to pin back or reshape ears will not produce a noticeable change in hearing.

Advanced techniques also are available to treat more severe ear problems. In those rare cases when a baby is born with no outer ear at all, it is possible for surgeons to construct a natural-looking outer ear. Reconstructive procedures also are used to repair ears damaged by traumatic injury or complications resulting from ear-piercing.

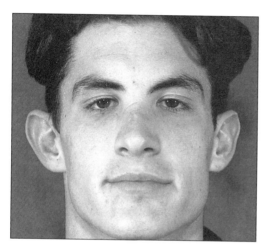 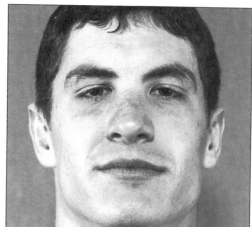

*Ear abnormalities that bring teasing and unkind comments often can be corrected with otoplasty.*

## NO NEED TO WAIT

Surgery to pin back protruding ears may be done as early as age five or six. By this time, the ear has achieved much of its adult size and is almost completely formed. The cartilage, however, is still soft and easily molded, making it possible to get good results.

Some people feel there may be an emotional benefit in having the surgery done during childhood, as Traci B. explains: "I wish I could have had my ears corrected when I was little. It's hard to grow up feeling different."

Because small children may have a higher risk of complications, many parents choose to defer surgery until the child is older. Although adult ear cartilage is less flexible than that of a child, otoplasty may be done successfully at any age. Joanne J. was past 40 at the time of her operation. "I wanted it all my life, and I finally was able to have it done," she states. "I just wish I had done it sooner."

A few otoplasty patients find that the cartilage doesn't stay back in its new position as well as desired. If a satisfactory improvement is not obtained, a second minor procedure may be recommended.

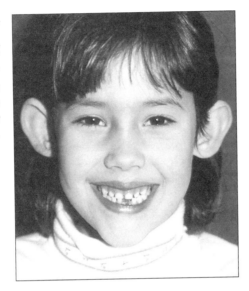
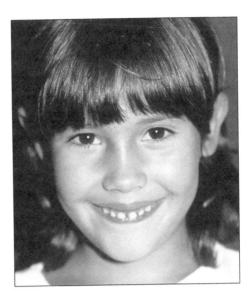

## HOW EAR SURGERY IS DONE

Ear surgery incisions are made behind the ear, where they are easily hidden in a natural crease *(see Figure 2)*. The surgeon removes excess skin and sculpts the cartilage, reducing the size of the ears and repositioning them closer to the head. Permanent sutures may be placed in the cartilage to secure its position and create natural-looking ear folds. The procedure typically lasts one to two hours.

Otoplasty may be performed in a hospital, an outpatient surgical facility, or in the surgeon's office depending on the age of the patient, the extent of the surgery, and the preference of the surgeon. Young children usually receive general anesthesia and may spend a night in the hospital. Adults typically have the procedure done with local anesthesia and intravenous sedation (twilight sleep).

*Figure 2
Ear surgery
incision*

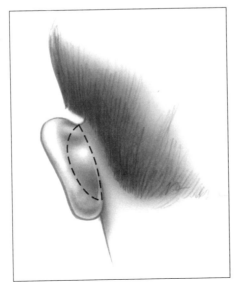

More complex reconstructive procedures may require several steps. Cartilage may be taken from another part of the body, such as the ribs, to construct or rebuild the outer ear. Tissue expanders may be used to stretch adjacent non-hair-bearing skin to form a covering for the ear.

## AFTER THE SURGERY

After ear surgery, a soft, padded bandage will be placed around your head to protect your ears and hold them in place. When this is removed, you may be advised to wear a stretchy headband or stocking cap for a week or so longer, especially at night.

"There wasn't much pain at first," Joanne J. recalls. "I guess I was still numb from the surgery. After that wore off, it was somewhat painful for a day or two, but not unbearable." Although most people report some discomfort, it is easily controlled with mild pain medication.

Most people go back to school or work within a week. "I had some bruising and swelling around my ears, but it went away quickly," says Todd B., who had his surgery on the first day of spring break in his senior year. "A week later I went back to school, and no one suspected a thing."

Few risks are involved in otoplasty. "For me, the worst part of it was going to sleep at night," Joanne notes. "I like to sleep on my side, and for the first two weeks I had to get used to sleeping on my back."

## A NEW START
Ear surgery can offer a real emotional boost in addition to its cosmetic benefits.

"My whole personality changed," Traci B. enthusiastically says. "I feel so free now! I can enjoy what I'm doing, and not worry about whether my ears will show. Before I spent hours arranging my hair. Now I just put it up and go. I'm even playing tennis—and I'm loving it."

"Having the surgery before going away to college really helped me," asserts Todd. "It gave me a fresh start. I feel a lot more confident than I used to, especially when going into unknown situations. I know I look good, and that makes me more sure of myself. I'm really glad I had this done."

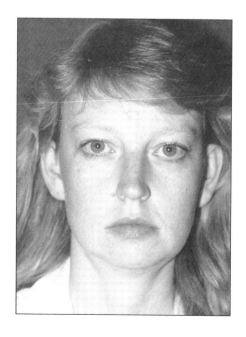
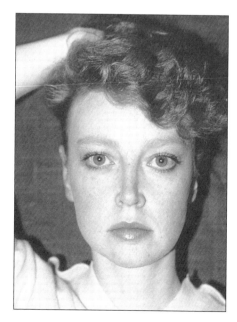

*Ear surgery can offer a real emotional boost, in addition to its cosmetic benefits.*

# *Repairing damaged ears*

It can happen in a moment—an unthinking move to brush back your hair while wearing dangling earwires, and suddenly your earlobe is torn. Accidents can also occur when an earring gets caught on clothing or an inquisitive child makes a playful grab at a pretty dangler. In some cities, muggers on the run have yanked earrings off unwary victims. When such painful mishaps occur, otoplasty techniques can restore looks.

One technique for repairing a torn earlobe involves cutting a small triangular notch at the bottom of the lobe. A matching flap is created from tissue on the other side of the tear, and the two wedges are fit together and stitched. This lets the bottom of the lobe heal smoothly, without pulling or dimpling.

Depending on the nature of the injury, your facial plastic surgeon may select another method for repairing a tear. Common methods are a straight-line closure and Z-plasty, which involves cutting a zig-zag through the tear.

Earlobes typically heal quickly and with minimal scarring. In most cases, the earlobe can be repierced six to 12 weeks after surgical reconstruction.

If you like to wear big earrings, it's a good idea to give your earlobes a rest periodically. Heavy earrings can cause an unsightly enlargement of the holes, weakening the lobes and increasing the risk of tearing.

And think carefully before deciding to have multiple holes made in your ears, particularly around the tops and sides. Piercing the cartilage is unwise, from a medical standpoint, because infection can develop and loss of cartilage may occur. Ears damaged in this way will need to be reconstructed surgically.

*Attention is drawn from the ears to the face when protruding ears are corrected with otoplasty.*

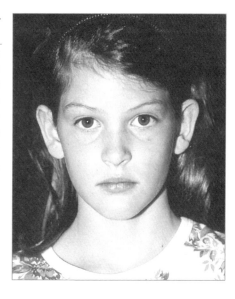
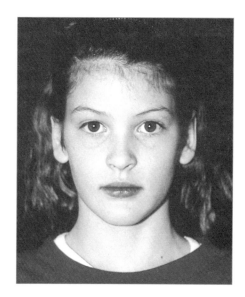

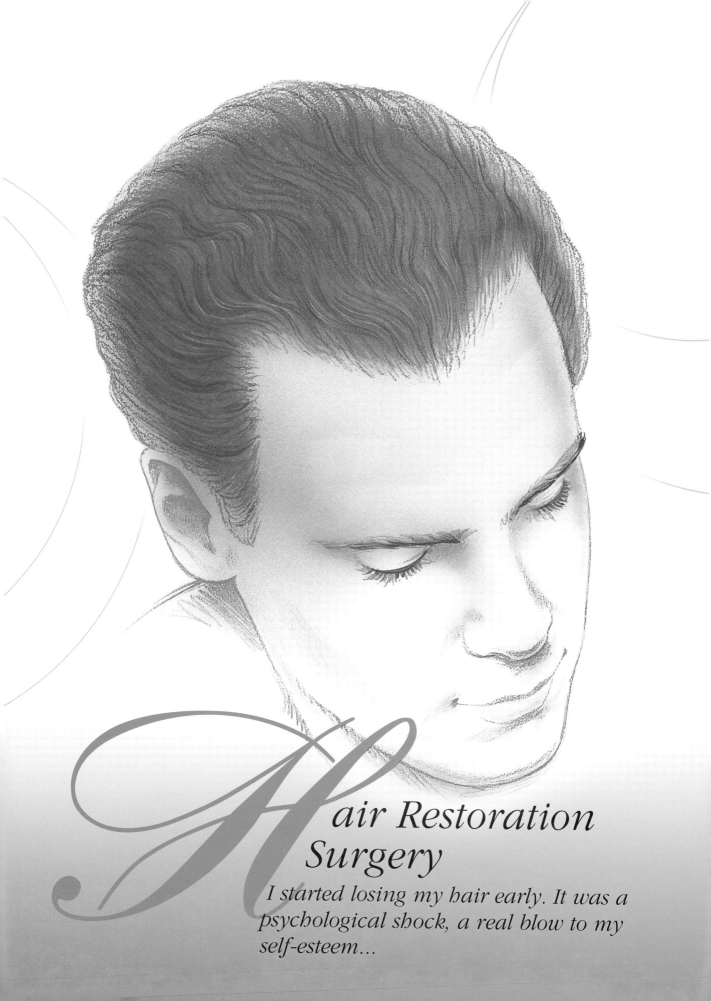

# Hair Restoration Surgery

*I started losing my hair early. It was a psychological shock, a real blow to my self-esteem...*

# Hair Restoration Surgery

*"I started losing my hair early. It was a psychological shock, a real blow to my self esteem. Then, when my wife left me for a younger-looking man, I took a long, hard look at myself, and I didn't like what I saw: an overweight guy who was going bald. I had been used to thinking of myself as a fairly attractive guy, but I didn't feel attractive any more. It was time for action. So I started a physical fitness program and began treatment for hair restoration. Now I look at least 10 years younger than I did before. It's made a tremendous difference in the way people relate to me—and in the way I feel about myself."*

■ *Bob E., age 41*

Most men will agree—losing your hair causes emotional distress. It's an experience, unfortunately, that nearly all men will share. In fact, if you are male and over 30, you probably already have looked in the mirror and bemoaned the thinning of your hairline. If you are very lucky, you may only have some thinning around the temples and at the crown. But for many men, growing older means growing balder—a bare spot at the crown and extensive hair loss over the front and top of the head. Doctors call this "male pattern baldness," and it's a fact of life for most men. In fact, two-thirds of all men experience a significant degree of hair loss.

Despite its pervasiveness, baldness is hardly seen as desirable. A number of studies have suggested that balding men tend to be viewed as less attractive, older, and less likely to be successful than their non-balding counterparts. Men may laugh about it—and who can escape baldness jokes?—but inside they feel self-conscious and helpless. Hair loss is just not funny when it happens to you.

8

*For many men, growing older means growing balder—a bare spot at the crown and extensive hair loss over the front and top of the head.*

# *Not for men only*

Everyone has heard of "male pattern baldness," but men aren't the only ones who suffer from hair loss. Irreversible hair loss can occur in men and women of all ages—and even in children. The loss may be inherited or traumatic.

Although women do not experience inherited hair loss as frequently as men, it does occur. In rare cases, women may experience permanent hair thinning after pregnancy. Some hairstyles can cause permanent bald spots, or acquired alopecia, when ponytails or barrettes are worn for years, putting stress on hair follicles. Thinning hair may be camouflaged by a woman's hairstyle up to a point, but a growing bald spot can be devastating to a woman's self-esteem.

Even more devastating—for anyone—are accidents or burns that destroy or damage large areas of the scalp, or even eyebrows. Permanent hair loss also can result from illness, exposure to drugs or other chemicals, and even for no known cause. Fortunately, facial plastic surgery offers a number of options to individuals who have suffered permanent hair loss for whatever reason.

When sufficient donor hair is available, transplantation is the easiest treatment for hair loss; however, it may not provide sufficient fullness for many women. Flap surgery and tissue expansion are often a better choice, particularly when hair loss results from a burn or scalp injury. When just a small area is affected, scalp reduction may solve the problem.

Careful evaluation is especially essential before any procedure is performed, because poorly done hair replacement procedures can lead to visible scars or unnatural patterns of baldness. A facial plastic surgeon with experience in reconstructive procedures and hair replacement surgery is best qualified to give advice on treating permanent hair loss.

*An automobile accident left this four-year-old girl with scarring and hair loss, which were reversed with tissue expansion and hair flap surgery.*

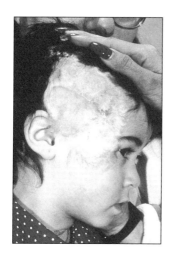
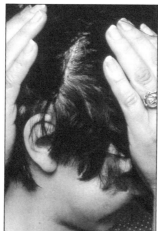
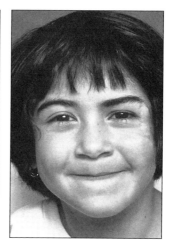

"I think hair is everything," comments Germaine Gomez. "I work out regularly to keep in shape, and losing my hair really bothered me. It wasn't that people treated me differently; it was just a personal feeling. I wanted to look as good as I felt—and I wanted my own hair."

For Germaine, the solution was a series of hair transplant procedures—one of several permanent solutions available for hair loss.

"I tried a drug treatment, but it didn't work for me," he says. "I didn't want a wig. Now I have my own hair, growing naturally. It's unbelievable how great it looks."

Facial plastic surgery offers several effective techniques for treating hair loss, including hair grafts, scalp flap surgery, and scalp reduction. One of these options—or a combination of methods—may be right for you.

## PATTERNS OF MALE BALDNESS

Before selecting an appropriate treatment for male pattern baldness, your surgeon will consider the extent of your hair loss, how your remaining hair is distributed, and your ultimate balding pattern. The most important thing to remember about male pattern baldness is that it is progressive. Therefore, treatment must take into account what is going to happen in the future.

*If you have avoided having hair transplant surgery, fearing it would give you a "pluggy" appearance, it may be time for you to give this method of hair restoration surgery another look.*

Whatever procedure is selected, the goal of hair replacement surgery is to give you a natural appearance that will look good for the rest of your life. It is important to identify your final balding pattern so that donor hair is not taken from any area that is programmed for future hair loss. Subsequent thinning of treated areas also must be considered. Keep in mind, however, that the precise extent of future hair loss cannot always be predicted accurately.

To help predict future hair loss, facial plastic surgeons have identified four types of balding patterns. Male pattern baldness usually begins at the front of the head with a receding hairline *(see Figure 1)*. It typically continues across the top of the scalp, and a bald spot may appear on the crown. In many men, these areas eventually meet, producing the classic

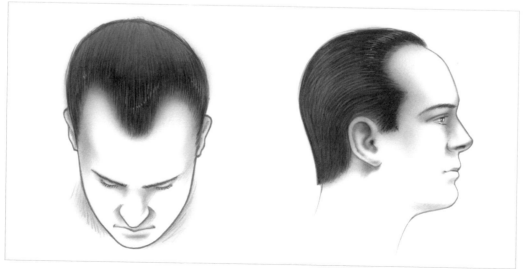

*Figure 1*
*Front baldness only*

▶
*Figure 2*
*Front to*
*crown baldness*

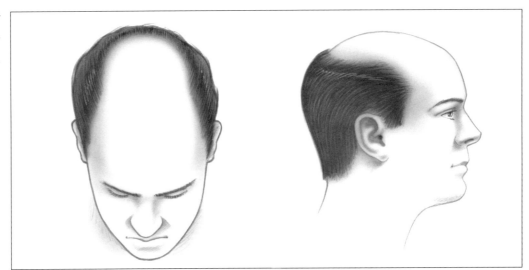

▶
*Figure 3*
*Front and*
*midscalp*
*baldness,*
*with no*
*thinning*
*of the crown*

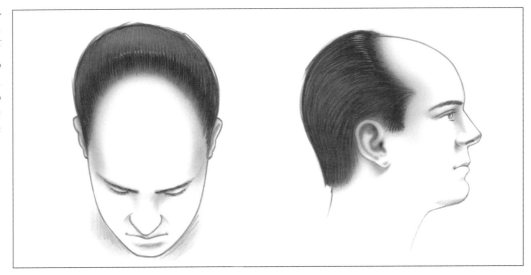

▶
*Figure 4*
*Crown*
*baldness*
*only*

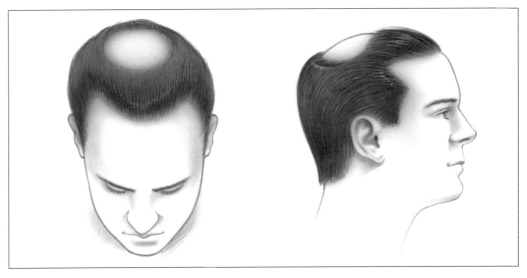

horseshoe-shaped rim of hair around the edge of the scalp *(see Figure 2)*. In other cases, the hair line recedes to the middle of the scalp, with little or no thinning at the crown *(see Figure 3)*. Rarely, a man will develop crown baldness only, with normal thickness in all other areas *(see Figure 4)*.

## TODAY'S HAIR GRAFTS

Hair grafting is the oldest method of surgical hair replacement, and it is still the most common. In one respect, it also can be considered the newest method because techniques have changed significantly in the past few years. In fact, if you have avoided having hair transplant surgery, fearing it would give you a "pluggy" appearance, it may be time for you to give this method of hair restoration surgery another look.

In the past, hair transplants were called "punch grafts," because the technique involved punching out little circles of hair-bearing skin about one-sixth inch in diameter from the back of the head and transplanting them in the bald area. The spacing of these circular "plugs" meant that hair would grow in little tufts, rather like doll's hair, necessitating careful styling to camouflage the effect.

Today, hair grafting is a more sophisticated technique, involving many more grafts of a much smaller size. The transplanted pieces of hair-bearing skin are called minigrafts or micrografts, according to their size. These tiny grafts provide better hair distribution and a more natural hairline. In fact, if you have had a hair transplant in the past that has a tufted appearance, you now may be able to have mini- and micrografts placed between the original plugs to refine your overall appearance.

Hair grafting is usually done under local anesthesia in the surgeon's office. You may be given intravenous sedation or an oral medication to help you relax, if you wish.

"I can't take pain," reports Bill H. "But I had no pain at all with my hair transplant procedures. The doctor used a local anesthetic, and I was awake the whole time, talking, watching

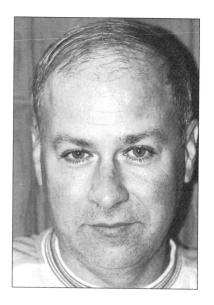
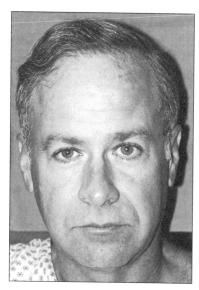

◄

*Transplanted grafts of hair-bearing skin produce new hair growth that is usually permanent.*

television, and drinking coffee. I could get up and walk around when I needed to stretch. Afterward, I put on a ball cap and drove home. I never needed any pain medication."

The most important step of a hair transplant is planning the procedure and designing an appropriate hairline for you. Your skin tone and hair color, as well as the availability of donor hair follicles, will help determine the coverage that can be achieved. The front should be treated first, because that is the area that is most visible. If enough donor hair follicles are available, you may have the crown done as well.

To do the procedure, the doctor first uses a fine, multi-bladed knife to cut strips of various widths from the donor site across the back of your head. These strips are cut into hundreds of individual grafts of different sizes. Each graft contains as many as five to nine hair follicles (for minigrafts) or as few as one or two hairs (for micrografts). The surgeon then transplants these into the bald area, after first removing a small piece of bald skin or making a tiny opening at the graft site. The grafts are held in place by the tiny drop of coagulated blood that forms at each transplant site—no adhesives or stitches are used.

Space is left around each graft in order to ensure an adequate blood supply for each newly transplanted hair follicle. The grafts are placed throughout the bald area in a pattern that mimics natural hair growth, with larger grafts placed in the center of the area to be treated and minigrafts filling the bulk of the space. Micrografts of one or two hair follicles are used along the hairline to give it a soft, natural look.

Grafts are done in several sessions spaced one to four months apart. At each session, additional grafts are placed in between the older ones until the desired density is obtained *(see Figure 5)*. Depending on the size of the area to be treated, you may need two to four

*Figure 5*
*Placement of grafts in recipient sites*

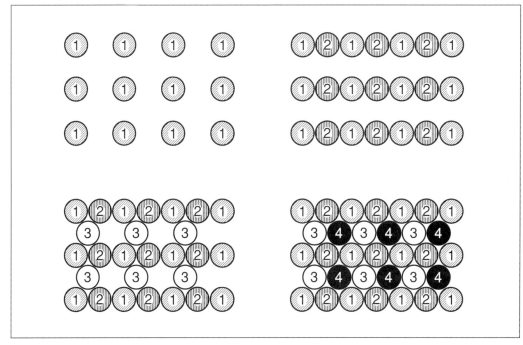

## Lasers for hair replacement?

Lasers are being used in all types of surgery today, including hair transplantation. Experts are still divided, however, on whether lasers enhance surgical results.

Some surgeons use a laser device instead of a scalpel to prepare the site where each graft is placed. The high-intensity laser beam vaporizes the skin, creating an opening that is slightly wider than a typical incision. The wider slit allows easier insertion of the graft, some doctors say, and the incision is completely bloodless. On the other hand, there is almost no bleeding during hair transplant surgery, and the little bit of blood at each graft site acts like a glue to secure the graft in place.

What about the results? Some studies suggest that grafts placed with lasers may grow in faster and thicker than those placed in the conventional way. Other studies have shown no real difference. Furthermore, the technology is still in its infancy and few surgeons are using it routinely.

"Lasers are just a tool," maintains one facial plastic surgeon. "The real key to good results is not the tool used to make the incision, but the skill and artistry of the surgeon."

*Micrografts of one or two hair follicles are used along the hairline to give it a soft, natural look.*

sessions, or more. Usually 300 to 500 grafts will be placed each time, although some surgeons may place as many as 1,500 in a single session.

Stitches placed along the donor site are completely hidden by your hair. Most patients return to work the following day. A tiny crust may form at the site of each graft; these fall off about two weeks after surgery. You will need to be careful about combing over the transplant site for about a week, but you should be able to shampoo gently three days after surgery. Stitches are removed at 10 days, and no other follow-up is normally needed.

The transplanted hair usually falls out within six weeks after surgery. This is no cause for concern—the hair follicles soon begin to produce new hair, which grows at the normal rate of about one-half inch per month. It takes a year or more to see the final results, but the new growth usually is permanent. Because grafts are taken only from an area that is not subject to male pattern baldness, the transplanted hair should continue to grow for the rest of your life.

"When I meet people I haven't seen in a long time, they can't believe it," says Bob E. "I tell people I had a transplant, and they're amazed. It looks completely natural."

## SCALP FLAP SURGERY

Scalp flap surgery is another method of hair replacement that can offer dramatic results for some people. It involves rotating strips of hair-bearing scalp from the side and back of the head to the front and top. In this way, scalp flap surgery can restore the hairline while maintaining normal hair density. Although it involves more extensive surgery than grafts, it provides immediate results.

*Source*
*of flaps*

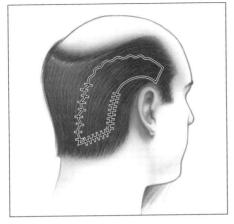

"My hair started thinning when I was in college," says Brian W., a 37-year-old sales representative for a publishing company. A friend told me about flap surgery, and I decided to look into it. The results were super. I now have the hairline that I had in high school."

Flap surgery begins with an evaluation of your baldness pattern to ensure that flaps can be taken from an area that will not be subject to hair loss. Then the surgeon designs your new hairline with your cooperation.

The procedure is done in three steps. During the first step, the surgeon marks a 1½-inch wide strip on the side of your head that is long enough to extend across the bald area. Care is taken to incorporate a blood vessel, called the superficial temporal artery, within the flap. Then incisions are made on the top and bottom of the strip, separating the flap from the surrounding skin. The incisions are closed immediately with sutures or surgical clips. This step, called a "delay," increases blood flow to the flap to ensure its continued health after it is rotated.

One week later, a second delay is performed. In this step, the surgeon extends the original incisions and cuts around the tail of the flap, once again closing the incision and leaving the upper end of the flap attached above the ear *(see Figure 6)*. Each delay procedure takes about 30 minutes, and afterward you may resume your ordinary activities.

"I actually called on clients the same afternoon," Brian recalls. "I went home and washed my hair and then went back to work. The incisions were not noticeable and caused little discomfort."

The third step is the rotation of the flap, which is done one week after the second delay. It may be done in a hospital or an office surgery center, usually under light general anesthesia. The surgeon lifts the flap, removes a corresponding strip of bald scalp, and rotates the flap into its new position. The hair-bearing skin surrounding the donor area is stretched and secured with stitches or surgical clips. The new hairline is sutured in a way that allows hair to grow through the scar, effectively camouflaging it.

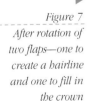

*After rotation of*
*two flaps—one to*
*create a hairline*
*and one to fill in*
*the crown*

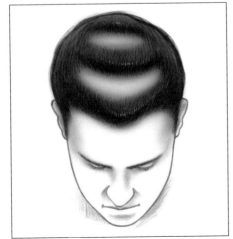

"After the rotation, I had to take it easy for about a week," says Brian. "I wore a turban-like bandage for a few days, but I could shampoo my hair about three days after surgery. The stitches were taken out a week or so later."

You may have some slight swelling or a feeling of tightness near the donor site for a few weeks after flap surgery. Pain is minimal, however, and most of it subsides within the first 24 hours.

Rotating the flap typically produces a slight bulge of scalp tissue at the hairline, where the flap is folded back on itself. This bump, called a "dog-ear," is removed in a minor procedure done about six weeks after the flap rotation.

The initial flap procedure restores your hairline and eliminates frontal baldness. Baldness over the top of the head may be corrected by a second flap procedure done at least three months later. The second flap is taken from the opposite side of the head and placed an inch or so behind the first one *(see Figure 7)*. The procedure is somewhat simpler because the hairline is not involved and the flap does not need to be rotated quite as far.

Scalp flap surgery reduces baldness immediately and yields a uniform thickness of hair that can be styled any way you wish. "My hair looks totally natural," Brian says. "This procedure was ideal for me. I'm delighted with the results."

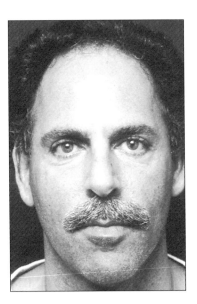 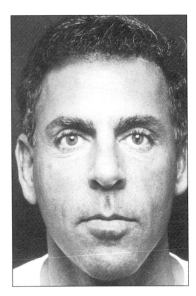

◄

*Frontal baldness can be eliminated with scalp flap surgery.*

## SCALP REDUCTION AND TISSUE EXPANDERS

In some individuals, surgery to reduce the size of the bald area may be recommended as part of the overall treatment plan. This procedure, called scalp reduction, usually does not eliminate baldness entirely, but it is often done in conjunction with hair transplantation or scalp flap surgery.

Scalp reduction may be done in the doctor's office under local anesthesia. Incisions are made in the scalp and a portion of bald skin is cut out *(see Figure 8)*. Then the incisions are closed and a dressing is applied. On the following day, the dressing is removed and you

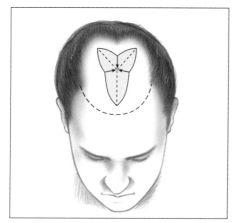

*Figure 8*
*Scalp reduction*
*incisions*

may resume most normal activities. Stitches are removed 10 to 14 days after surgery. Additional reduction procedures may be performed 12 weeks apart. This gives the scalp time to regain its normal elasticity.

Patients with tight scalps or an inadequate amount of donor hair may benefit from a procedure called tissue expansion. This technique stretches the skin gradually by means of a balloon-like device implanted under a hair-bearing portion of the scalp. Sterile salt water is injected into each balloon twice a week for six to eight weeks. This is done in the doctor's office, or a willing family member may be trained to do the injections. When the expansion is complete, the balloon is removed, an area of bald scalp is cut away, and a scalp reduction or flap procedure is completed. If necessary, mini- or micrografts may be done later to cover the scar and fill any bald area that remains.

## WHICH HAIR RESTORATION PROCEDURE IS FOR YOU?

Each hair restoration method has advantages and limitations. Grafts, for instance, require several sessions, and it may take one to two years to see the finished results. Full coverage may be difficult to achieve if you have extensive baldness or a marked contrast between your hair and skin color. On the plus side, hair grafting is the simplest and most appealing method of hair restoration, and it is widely available. It is appropriate for most men experiencing hair loss, and it can provide excellent results.

Flap surgery can restore a full hairline almost instantly, but it involves more extensive surgery. Some individuals—for example, heavy smokers and others who may have problems with blood circulation—may not be good candidates for the procedure. It may be difficult to find a surgeon who has the appropriate training and experience. Scalp reduction works best in patients who have a fairly elastic scalp skin. Excessive tissue expansion or scalp reduction may cause scarring, problems with hair growth patterns, or thinning of the hairline around the sides and back of the head.

The best procedure for you depends on many factors, including your age, state of health, skin quality and elasticity, hair color, skin tone, the extent of your baldness, and the likelihood of future hair loss. In some cases, a combination of procedures may be needed to provide the best results. Your facial plastic surgeon can help you explore the issues involved and determine which procedures may be best for you.

# No easy answers

Hair restoration is a multi-million dollar business today. Many of the treatments touted, however, do little to solve the problem of hair loss. The only permanent solution is surgery.

Numerous shampoos, conditioners, nutritional supplements, and herbal preparations claim to "unclog" hair follicles, increase blood flow to the scalp, or provide nutrients needed for hair growth. Male pattern baldness is not caused by poor hygiene or nutrition, however; such products do not promote hair growth.

Only one drug, minoxidil, is known to stimulate new hair growth. Originally introduced as a blood pressure medication, this drug has been available since 1988 in a form that can be applied directly to the scalp. Minoxidil does not work for everyone, however. In some people, it produces only scanty growth or none at all. In others, it only seems to slow the rate of balding. It also must be used indefinitely by those who find it helpful. Regrown hair falls out when the drug is discontinued. Finasteride, a drug used to treat prostate enlargement, seems to slow down the rate of hair loss. Although it does not stimulate new growth, it may have some potential for treating hair loss.

Hairpieces are a common solution to the problem of hair loss. Although a hairpiece can give the appearance of a full head of hair instantly, a good quality one is expensive. Hairpieces must be cleaned regularly, and they need to be replaced every few years.

Techniques for securing hairpieces to the scalp have included adhesives, surgical sutures, and even snaps permanently implanted in the scalp. Adhesives are relatively safe, but they sometimes cause irritation or an unpleasant odor. Surgical sutures and other devices implanted into the scalp can cause infection and other problems, and are illegal in some states.

Hair weaving is a method of attaching a hairpiece to existing hair. Bonding, another non-surgical approach, involves gluing or sewing replacement hair to your existing hair, giving the appearance of greater fullness. These arrangements require regular service as your natural hair grows, and over time, the cost can become considerable. They also can damage your existing hair.

Many people find that the increased self-confidence and sense of well-being that result from surgical hair replacement make it a worthwhile investment.

*Many people find that the increased self-confidence and sense of well-being that result from surgical hair replacement make it a worthwhile investment.*

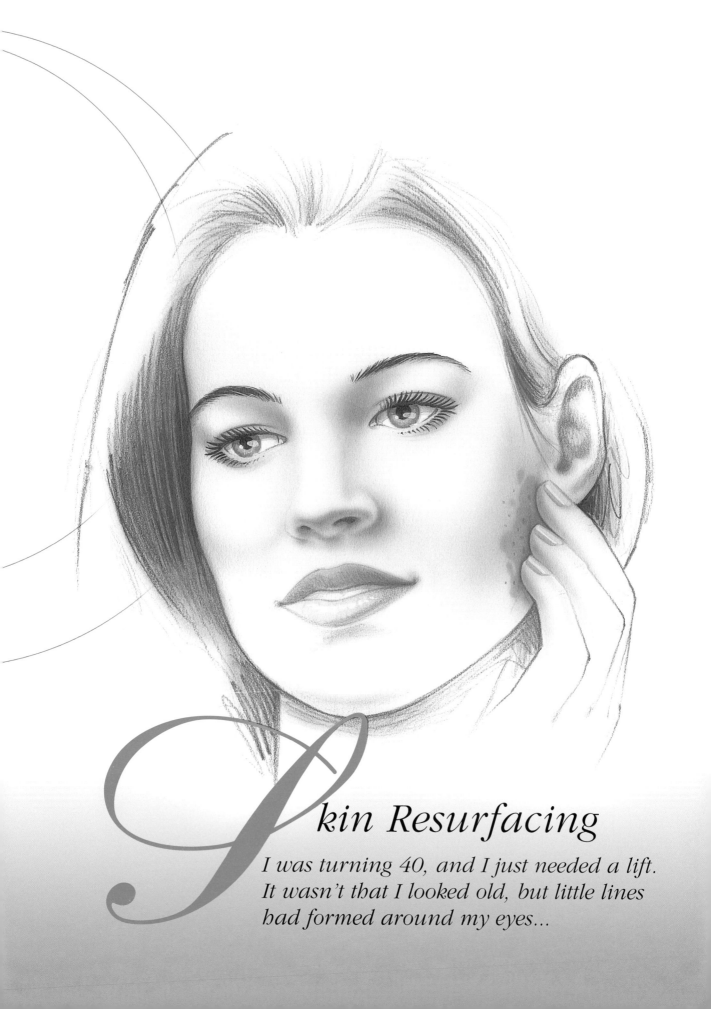

# Skin Resurfacing

*I was turning 40, and I just needed a lift.
It wasn't that I looked old, but little lines
had formed around my eyes...*

# Skin Resurfacing

*"I was turning 40, and I just needed a lift. It wasn't that I looked old, but little lines had formed around my eyes, and the creases from either side of my nose to the corners of my mouth were growing more pronounced. Those lines made me look like "Deputy Dawg," and they drove me crazy. About the time I realized that my regular workouts weren't going to reverse these signs of aging, I became aware of laser resurfacing. Now, after full-face resurfacing, the lines are much less noticeable, and my skin looks young and fresh again. It's just what I needed to get me over the hump of turning 40."*

■ *Terri Speck, age 40*

Smooth, fresh, unblemished skin—it's what everyone wants. Women have always prized a clear complexion, with skin that is unwrinkled, even-toned, and free from bumps or spots. Men are a little more tolerant of what has been termed "the rugged look," but they too want healthy, youthful-looking skin.

In days gone by, women protected their milk-white complexions with big bonnets and parasols. Today, they enjoy a more active outdoor lifestyle, wearing clothes that leave limbs free to move—and skin exposed to the elements. Unfortunately, great-great grandma was right: Unprotected skin ages more rapidly.

"I loved being tanned," says Terri Speck, recalling her sun-worshiping days. Like thousands of other one-time sun-bronzed beauties, she learned the hard way that sun exposure causes premature wrinkling and a weathered appearance. Since Terri had her skin resurfaced, she avoids the sun. "Now I want to protect my new complexion," she says.

The sun is not the only culprit, of course. Time inevitably brings lines and wrinkles to the

9

*A number of techniques are available today that enable facial plastic surgeons to treat a wider range of skin problems than ever before.*

faces of the most dedicated sunblock users. For others, skin quality is marred by heredity and environmental factors that cause unsightly blotches, acne scars, freckles, precancerous lesions, and other blemishes—or more permanent lesions, such as café au lait spots, strawberry birthmarks, and spider veins. One form of skin discoloration—tattoos—is the result of a personal choice that many people later regret.

*Skin resurfacing removes the epidermis and penetrates into the papillary dermis, which responds by producing new collagen.*

Whatever their origin, skin problems can be the source of great emotional pain, as June B. relates: "I didn't have much trouble with acne as a teenager, but my face bloomed in college," she says. "The acne never quite went away, and then I really broke out badly when I was pregnant with my first child. Nothing helped, and I became very self-conscious about my skin. All I wanted was to find some way to make it better, so I could feel good about myself again."

Fortunately, a number of techniques are available today that enable facial plastic surgeons to treat a wider range of skin problems than ever before. The technique that is right for you will depend on many factors, including what type of problem you have, its severity, your skin type, your state of health, and your surgeon's experience with successfully treating problems like yours with various techniques. In some cases, a combination of techniques and multiple treatments may be recommended.

## WHAT IS SKIN RESURFACING, AND HOW DOES IT WORK?

All techniques—from more traditional chemical peels and facial sanding to the latest laser treatments—involve resurfacing the skin. To picture how resurfacing works, imagine an old table covered with multiple coats of paint, its surface bumpy and wrinkled from years of hard use. If you coat it with a good furniture stripper, the old paint will bubble up so that it can be wiped away—revealing the beautiful wood grain underneath. Or, you might sand the table to remove the damaged surface and smooth out dents and imperfections.

▼ *Figure 1*
*Layers of the skin:*
*A. Epidermis;*
*B. Papillary dermis;*
*C. Reticular dermis*

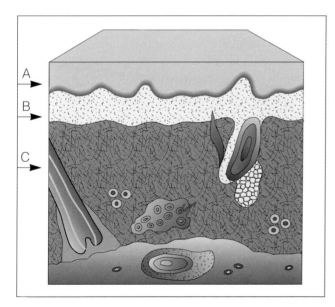

Skin resurfacing follows the same principle: The damaged upper layers of the skin are removed to allow new, undamaged skin to grow in its place.

To understand more precisely what happens, it is helpful to know that the skin is made up of two layers: an outer layer called the epidermis and a deeper layer called the dermis. The dermis is composed mostly of long fibers of collagen, the normal protein of the skin. Under a microscope, these fibers look like spaghetti thrown on a table— long, thin strands with no organized pattern. The dermis itself has two levels: the upper "papillary dermis" and the deeper "reticular dermis" *(see Figure 1).*

Superficial wrinkles, freckles, and minor pigmentation problems generally originate in the lower level of the epidermis and extend beyond it into the upper layer of the dermis. Skin resurfacing removes the epidermis and penetrates into the papillary dermis, which responds by producing new collagen. Collagen fibers tend to become shorter, thicker, and more organized as the dermis heals, thus, skin resurfacing not only eliminates many fine lines and blemishes, it also refines the texture of the skin. The process takes several months, so improvement may continue to be seen for about one year after the skin is resurfaced.

Scars and deep wrinkles typically involve the reticular dermis. Skin resurfacing procedures do not penetrate this deeply, because any injury to the reticular dermis is likely to cause scarring. This explains why scars and wrinkles are improved by skin resurfacing, but not entirely eliminated.

## CHEMICAL PEELING

Many facial plastic surgeons resurface the skin with an acid solution that peels the top layers and allows smoother, regenerated skin to emerge. Chemical peeling is an effective treatment for wrinkles caused by sun damage, mild scarring, and certain types of acne. Age spots, blotches, and dull skin tone also may be improved through chemical peeling.

Different types of solutions are used, depending on the severity of the problem, to provide a peel that is superficial, medium, or deep. In general, deeper peels give better and more long-lasting results. Mild peels offer a quicker recovery time, but may not provide as dramatic an improvement.

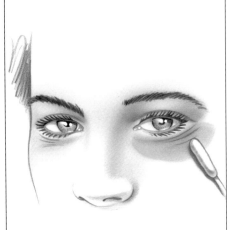

*Figure 2*
*Chemical peel*

Chemical peeling is usually done in the surgeon's office. Small areas may be done without anesthesia, but light sedation usually is recommended for a full face peel.

Before the procedure, your skin is thoroughly cleansed with an antiseptic solution that removes facial oils and prepares your skin for deep penetration. Then the surgeon applies the chemical solution with an applicator *(see Figure 2)*. You will notice a burning sensation as the chemical is applied, which may intensify over 20 to 30 minutes. Most people compare the pain to a mild to moderate sunburn. Mild pain relievers are given to control discomfort.

After the chemical peel is completed, a cream or antibiotic ointment may be applied to your face to protect the surface and keep it moist. In about 10 days, you will see delicate pink skin that appears smoother and tighter than before. Your face will continue to be red for several weeks afterward, but this can be camouflaged with makeup. Most people regain their normal skin tone within six to eight weeks.

For many people, chemical peeling is the first step to maintaining a youthful appearance.

"I was only 40, and I didn't need a facelift yet," is how one patient puts it. "The peeling procedure brightened my complexion, softened the deep lines around my mouth, and made the little smile wrinkles around my eyes virtually unnoticeable."

For others, the procedure is the "icing on the cake" following more extensive surgery.

"I was 44 and starting to notice a little fold in my upper lids that hadn't been there before, and some tiny lines under my eyes," recalls Gloria M. Like many people who seek eyelid surgery —or facelifts or browlifts—she was pleased to find that surgery would tighten sagging muscles and remove excess skin, but was surprised to learn that it could not smooth out little lines and wrinkles. After a medium-strength peel around her eyes, "the lines were gone," she says. "The peel was easier than the eyelid surgery, and it made such a difference."

*Chemical peeling can smooth out lines and wrinkles after a facelift tightens the skin and underlying tissue.*

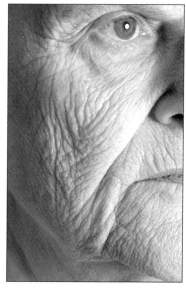
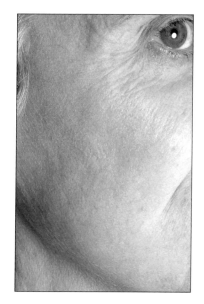
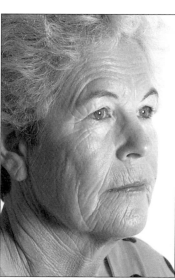
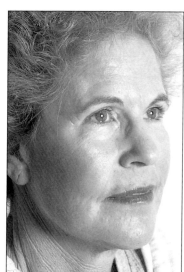

# Types of chemical peels

Chemical peels range from very superficial to deep, depending on the chemical used. Four types of chemical peels are used on the face. They include:

**Glycolic acid.** A natural substance derived from sugar cane, glycolic acid stimulates the production of collagen and thickens the dermis. Useful for treating minor wrinkles, clogged pores, and recurrent acne, it may be done by a facial plastic surgeon or a trained medical assistant working under the doctor's supervision. Except for a slight pinkening of the skin, there are no after-effects or discomfort. Glycolic acid treatments may be repeated at regular intervals, to improve and maintain the skin texture.

**Salicylic acid.** This mild chemical is sometimes used for superficial facial peels. Because it does not penetrate very deeply, it is ineffective against deep wrinkles. Superficial peels offer some improvement in skin tone and texture, but the results are considered temporary.

**Trichloroacetic acid (TCA).** This medium-strength chemical provides better results than superficial chemical peels. It is available in varying concentrations, which the surgeon can select to provide greater or lesser degrees of penetration depending on the nature of the problem. Healing time is generally shorter than that required after a phenol peel.

**Phenol.** The deepest type of chemical peel available, phenol peels often produce dramatic results that last for years. Phenol peels may be used to treat weathered skin, deep lines and wrinkles, and other types of facial blemishes.

*For many people, chemical peeling is the first step to maintaining a youthful appearance.*

One surgeon compares peels to ironing a garment after alterations: "A tailor can alter a suit to remove excess fabric and make it fit properly," he explains, "but it won't look right until he steams it to smooth out the wrinkles."

## DERMABRASION

To treat deeper scars and wrinkles, raised scar tissue, and other skin conditions, your surgeon may recommend dermabrasion, a facial sanding technique. Dermabrasion also is used to treat some severe cases of cystic acne that have failed to respond to other medical treatment. In dermabrasion, the top layers of skin are "sanded" off with a high-speed rotating brush or a diamond-coated wheel.

Before the dermabrasion procedure, you may be given a mild sedative intravenously. The area to be treated is thoroughly cleansed and then treated with a spray that freezes the top layer of skin, numbing the area and preparing the skin for the sanding procedure. Local anesthetics also may be used.

The surgeon uses the rotating abrasive instrument to remove the upper layers of skin and improve irregularities in the skin surface. A variety of tools may be used, depending on the problem being treated. For example, a pear-shaped tip is ideal for treating wrinkles around the base of the nose; a bullet-shaped tip may be used to focus on small spots or lesions. After the dermabrasion is complete, a soothing ointment and dressing are applied.

Immediately after dermabrasion, the treated area is raw and may ooze a yellowish fluid. Swelling peaks on the second to third day after dermabrasion and then starts to subside. Some patients experience throbbing or stinging during the first 24 hours. Any discomfort can be controlled with a mild pain reliever and ice compresses.

It is important to keep the treated area moist until the new skin appears, usually in about 10 days. The new skin is pink at first and gradually assumes a normal appearance within eight to 12 weeks. Makeup may be applied as soon as the skin is healed, and most people can return to work after one to two weeks.

## LASER SKIN RESURFACING

Another method of resurfacing the skin is by means of a device called the carbon dioxide ($CO_2$) laser. The $CO_2$ laser emits a colorless infrared light that vaporizes the top layer of skin instantly with no bleeding and little trauma to the surrounding tissue. The laser can be used with great precision, even in areas that cannot be treated safely with dermabrasion or chemical peeling. If necessary, the surgeon can make repeated passes in problem areas, shaving the skin down to a uniform level.

Laser resurfacing using the $CO_2$ device can correct a variety of problems, including wrinkles caused by excess sun exposure, "smile lines" and "crow's feet," and acne scarring. It also is effective for treating rhinophyma, a thickening of the nasal skin associated with enlarged oil glands; localized skin growths; and precancerous lesions that often occur on the lower lip.

Laser resurfacing (or "laserbrasion," as some surgeons call it) usually is done with local anesthesia. Light sedation may be recommended if a large area is to be treated.

"I was given an intravenous medication to help me relax, and the doctor used an anesthetic to numb my entire face," recalls Terri Speck. "I was awake during the entire procedure and I was actually talking part of the time. It was uncomfortable, but not unbearable."

*Laser resurfacing can minimize wrinkles caused by overexposure to the sun.*

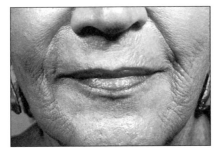
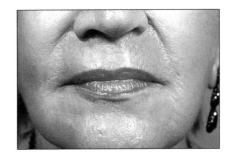

# Treating deeper skin problems

Although many surface skin lesions may be effectively treated through chemical peeling or dermabrasion, it is the advent of laser technology that has made possible the improvement of deeper facial blemishes that could not be treated effectively in the past. Various types of birthmarks, wart-like growths, spider veins, tattoos, and skin conditions like rosacea all may be treated successfully by lasers. Even infants and young children may be treated safely, thus minimizing some of the emotional trauma associated with disfiguring facial birthmarks.

Laser beams are generated by passing light through a gas-filled tube. The light energy is stimulated by electric current or radio waves and amplified by mirrors placed in the tube to produce an intense beam of light with special properties. The type of gas used determines the wavelength (or color) of the laser beam; the wavelength, in turn, determines the effect the beam has on the skin tissue.

The $CO_2$ laser emits a colorless infrared light that is absorbed by water-containing tissue, such as the skin. If highly focused, a $CO_2$ beam can cut through the skin and instantly seal off blood vessels. A diffused (unfocused), pulsed $CO_2$ laser beam vaporizes the top layer of skin without penetrating deeply into the underlying tissue. It is used for skin resurfacing and for treating warts, superficial birthmarks and tumors, and certain precancerous skin lesions.

Argon gas produces a blue-green light that is absorbed by hemoglobin, the red pigment found in blood cells. This allows the argon laser beam to penetrate the skin without damaging it. The laser energy heats the underlying blood vessels, effectively destroying them. The argon laser, therefore, is used to treat blemishes caused by abnormal blood vessels, such as port wine stains and strawberry marks.

A third type of laser, the flash-pumped dye laser, uses organic dye to produce laser beams in various colors, such as red, yellow, or green. It may be tuned to adjust the color of the beam, making it a versatile tool for treating a variety of lesions. Green light energy is used to treat oversized freckles, liver spots, and café au lait spots. Yellow light is absorbed best by red pigment, making it effective against red birthmarks, rosacea, and red-nose syndrome.

The Q-switched YAG (yttrium aluminum garnet) laser delivers extremely short, high-energy pulses of laser energy that are capable of very deep penetration. The YAG laser can remove tattoos without cutting or scarring, by breaking up the large globules of ink into small bits that can be carried away by the body's normal defense mechanism. It also is useful for treating deep vascular and pigmented lesions.

Large blemishes may require repeated treatments every six to eight weeks over a period of 12 to 18 months. Most blemishes can be significantly reduced, and some actually can be eliminated.

*The laser can be used with great precision, even in areas that cannot be treated safely with dermabrasion or chemical peeling.*

The laser resurfacing procedure takes about 30 minutes to an hour, depending on how much area is covered. Afterward you can go home with detailed instructions on how to care for the resurfaced area. You should expect considerable swelling, but most patients report only mild discomfort.

"Right after the procedure, my face was puffed up like a little round bear's," Terri remembers. "It was red and felt tight and somewhat raw. I took one of the pain pills the doctor had given me that night, but that was all."

*It is important to avoid sun exposure after any skin resurfacing procedure, because the new skin is fragile and easily damaged. Wear a wide-brimmed hat and apply a sunscreen lotion to protect your face whenever you plan to be outdoors.*

"Like a Sumo wrestler" is how 72-year-old Ronnie Lazar describes her appearance right after her resurfacing procedure. "It was not painful, just uncomfortable," she insists, "but it was well worth it to look so much better." Her laser resurfacing took place six months after a facelift, and the combination was clearly successful. "Just recently, I had to show identification to prove I was entitled to a senior citizen discount!"

Like these patients, your face will appear quite red for the first week or two. Then new, pink skin that is smoother and finer begins to emerge. It takes several months for all the redness to fade completely, but makeup may be used to camouflage it after a week or so. Most people return to work after 10 days to two weeks.

"I took 11 days off," recalls Terri. "My face was still red and a little swollen when I went back, but it didn't bother me. People probably thought I had a slight rash. It faded gradually over time, and it took months for the swelling to completely disappear."

## CARING FOR YOUR SKIN AFTER RESURFACING

Because the outer layer of skin is removed in a skin resurfacing procedure, it is essential to protect the surface and keep it moist while the area is healing. Your surgeon will give you detailed instructions on how to care for the treated area. You should follow these instructions carefully to minimize the formation of crusts and promote rapid healing.

"The worst part of the procedure for me was washing my face and seeing the dead skin slough off," says Terri. "I followed the doctor's instructions carefully, though, putting ointment on it regularly so scabs wouldn't form. It didn't last long—and my new skin looked so much better, it was worth the little bit of work."

Healing regimens vary depending on the size of the area treated, the method of skin resurfacing used, and your surgeon's preference. Many surgeons cover the abraded area with an occlusive dressing—a thin, soft material that clings tightly to the area and keeps air out—combined with a hydroactive gel that provides the proper physiologic moisture on the exposed surface. Others use a light gauze dressing, or none at all, along with regular applications of an antibiotic ointment or a moisturizing cream. Some surgeons prefer ordinary vegetable shortening or petroleum jelly.

Your surgeon may instruct you to wash your face several times a day to facilitate the sloughing of dead skin. Frequent showering may be recommended to float the crusts away and reduce any discomfort you may feel, or you might be advised to spray your face with water at specified intervals using a clean spray bottle.

It is important to avoid sun exposure after any skin resurfacing procedure, because the new skin is fragile and easily damaged. Wear a wide-brimmed hat and apply a sunscreen lotion (at least SPF 15) to protect your face whenever you plan to be outdoors. This is important both to prevent discoloration of the treated area and to keep your new skin looking its best.

"Sun exposure is what gave me those wrinkles," Terri comments. "I don't want them back, so I always use a sunblock now."

## CHANGES IN SKIN COLOR

Skin resurfacing can affect the skin color in some people, often causing it to become somewhat lighter. The decision to have a skin resurfacing procedure should be made with this in mind, as the change generally is permanent. For this reason, skin resurfacing may not be advisable for people with dark complexions.

More rarely, skin resurfacing may lead to darkened skin tone or uneven patches in the treated area. This may be treated with a bleaching agent if it occurs. Be sure to tell your surgeon if there is any family history of abnormal scarring or pigmentation problems.

For some people, pigment changes may be a desirable effect of skin resurfacing. After surgery to remove a tennis ball-sized tumor from his cheek, John M. needed extensive facial reconstruction. "The surgeon took a flap—complete with nerves and blood supply—from my arm to close the hole in my face," he explains. "When it healed, it was a darker color than the rest of my skin." John's surgeon suggested dermabrasion as a possible solution. "It was a risk because the skin-lightening effects of the procedure aren't predictable," John says, "but it worked—the discolored area is smaller and less noticeable now."

Ronnie Lazar was delighted with her new, lighter skin tone. "For years, I worked at tanning my face," she recalls. "At age 70, it was full of freckles and brown age spots. Skin resurfacing took away the wrinkles and restored my complexion. I have lovely skin now."

# *Birthmark or blemish—What is it?*

Nearly everyone is familiar with the small, dark moles commonly referred to as "beauty marks." These are simply deposits of melanin, the brown pigment found in the skin. There are many other types of skin blemishes as well. Some may be present at birth; others develop later in life. All are treatable by some resurfacing technique.

Here are some of the common type of skin blemishes:

**Hemangiomas**, the bumpy, red blemishes commonly called strawberry marks, actually are benign tumors of the capillary blood vessels. They typically appear during the first few months of life, grow rapidly for a time and then shrink gradually, often disappearing altogether.

**Port wine stains** are smooth areas of red or brown discoloration caused by abnormally enlarged blood vessels under the skin. Visible at birth, they enlarge as the child grows and are permanent unless treated.

**Café au lait spots** are smooth, light brown birthmarks caused by an excess of melanin.

**Lentigines**, also called age spots or liver spots, are oversized freckles. They tend to appear in older individuals, sometimes as a result of excessive sun exposure.

**Telangiectases**, or spider veins, are tiny, threadlike blood vessels that sometimes appear just beneath the skin surface, usually on the cheeks or nose.

**Rosacea** is a condition characterized by small, reddish bumps on the face, generally occurring in middle age.

**Rhinophyma**, or red-nose syndrome, is a severe form of rosacea that affects the nose. It is characterized by enlarged oil glands and a gradual thickening of the nasal skin that ultimately leads to enlargement of the nose itself.

**Seborrheic keratoses** are warty thickenings that may appear in middle age.

**Actinic keratoses** are patches of rough, reddish skin that sometimes develop after prolonged sun exposure, particularly in fair-skinned people.

**Xanthelasma** refers to small, elevated, yellowish growths that generally occur on the eyelids.

**Dermatosis papulosa nigra** is characterized by multiple raised, brown bumps on the upper cheeks near the eyes. It occurs most often in black and Asian individuals.

**Syringomas** are skin-colored growths that may develop on or near the lower eyelids or along the side of the nose.

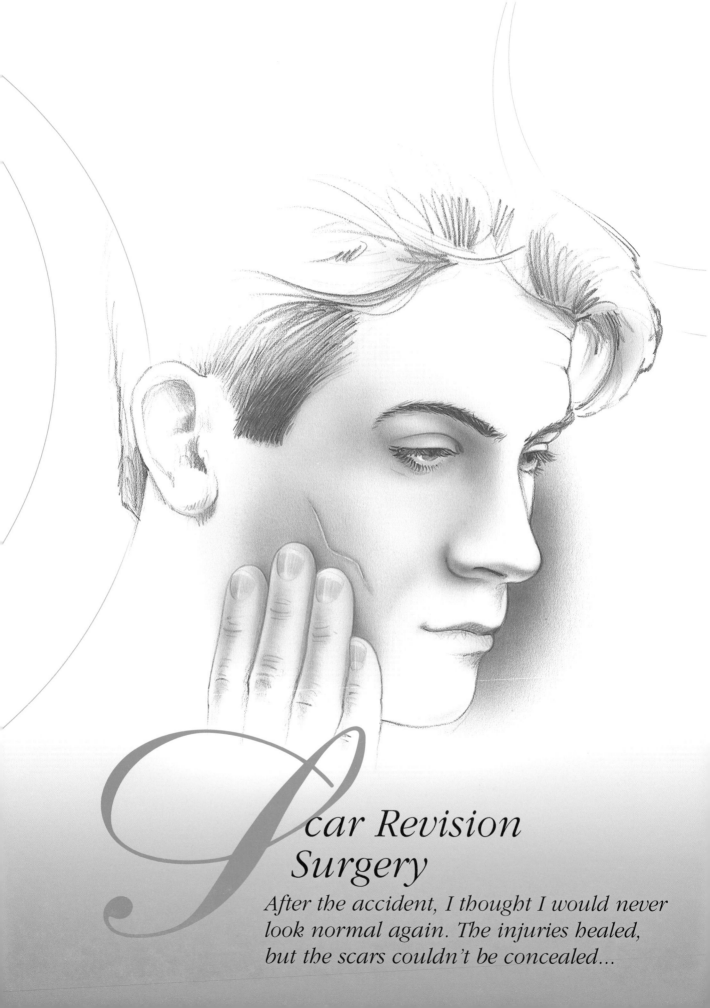

# Scar Revision Surgery

*After the accident, I thought I would never
look normal again. The injuries healed,
but the scars couldn't be concealed...*

# $\mathcal{S}$car Revision Surgery

*"After the accident, I thought I would never look normal again. The injuries healed, but the scars couldn't be concealed with makeup. People stared at me, and it bothered me to look the way I did. Now, after three revision procedures, I look much better. The scars are not completely gone, but I feel much better about the way I look. It helped me to put the accident behind me."*

■ *Laura G., age 34*

■ An unsightly facial scar can be devastating to your self-image—ask anyone who has had to live with one.

"It was very disturbing to me," says Shirley B., age 52, of the ragged scar stretching from her cheekbone to her chin. The victim of an assault, Shirley received prompt treatment of her injury, but a scar remained. "It really looked bad," she recalls. "I tried to cover it, but makeup didn't help. It made me feel terrible."

A disfiguring scar, as Shirley and Laura learned, also serves as an ever-present reminder of the traumatic experience that caused it. Even a scar that did not result from a traumatic event can cause emotional distress. Fortunately, much can be done to make scars less visible.

Surgery to improve the appearance of a scar is called scar revision surgery. A variety of techniques may be used, and often it is necessary to use more than one procedure in sequence. Scar revision procedures cannot eliminate scars entirely. The goal of surgery is to convert the scar into one that is less noticeable. It may be possible to make the scar smaller, to move it to a location where it is more easily hidden, or to change it in a way

10
- - - - - - - - - - -
*A disfiguring scar also serves as an ever-present reminder of the traumatic experience that caused it.*

that makes it less likely to attract attention. No matter how bad a scar looks, it usually can be made to look better.

## HOW SCARS FORM

Any time the deeper layers of skin are cut or torn, a scar results. Accidents, surgery, burns, or acne all can leave facial scars behind. Scars are permanent, but most scars fade gradually, eventually becoming nearly unnoticeable.

▶

*Scar revision surgery can improve the emotional as well as physical scars that result from a violent assault.*

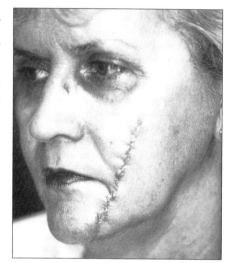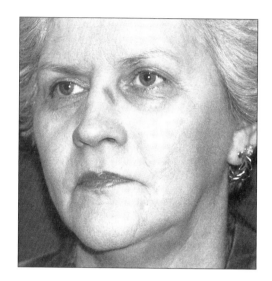

It is often difficult, right after an injury occurs, to predict what the final appearance of a scar will be. Scars tend to look worst during the early stages of healing. At first, tiny new blood vessels generally form around an injury to help speed the healing process. This causes the new scar to look red and noticeable. Next, collagen fibers begin to be laid down, giving the scar a raised or lumpy appearance. After about six weeks, most scars begin to shrink and soften—a process that may continue for up to two years.

*No matter how bad a scar looks, it usually can be made to look better.*

Some facial scars, however, do not improve with time. Severe burn scars, for example, often have a puckered appearance that time does not diminish. Acne may leave deep pits in the skin. Other scars, rather than shrinking, grow abnormally, forming hypertrophic scars. Keloids, a type of hypertrophic scar that results from an overproduction of collagen, continue growing beyond the margins of the original wound. Even a small scar may draw unwanted attention if it cuts across the face's natural creases and contours, and any scar that is unusually large, uneven, or differently colored may be nearly impossible to camouflage with makeup.

Some scars actually interfere with the normal function of facial features. A scar that contracts as it heals may restrict the movement of muscles and tendons or pull the lip or eyelid into an unnatural position.

It takes from six months to two years for a scar to reach the stage at which no further change will occur. The final appearance of the scar depends on your own ability to heal.

Some people have a tendency to scar more easily than others. Children, because of their ability to grow new cells, may develop larger and more visible scars that take a longer time to mature. Older people may heal with less scarring, and their scars may reach maturity somewhat faster.

*Scars tend to look worst during the early stages of healing.*

It is not possible to prevent scarring, even with the best of care. Ideally, facial injuries should be treated by a facial plastic surgeon, although this is not always possible. Even when initial treatment is done with the greatest of care, however, scar revision surgery may be needed later.

"A facial plastic surgeon was called into the emergency room to take care of my face," says Laura. "He did a good job, but he knew I would need scar revision later."

It's usually best to wait until a scar is mature before attempting scar revision surgery. It is wise, though, to consult a facial plastic surgeon soon after an injury occurs. The surgeon can ensure that the wound is closed in the best way possible, observe the scar in its early stages of healing, take photographs during the healing process, and plan what can be done later.

## SCAR REVISION TECHNIQUES

Scar revision surgery may involve one procedure, or it may require a series of procedures carried out over time.

Often, the easiest way to treat a scar is simply to excise it, or cut it out. In this way, a wide or lumpy scar may be replaced with a smaller, neater scar. This technique is sometimes used on hypertrophic scars.

A related technique, serial excision, is used to remove a large scar over a period of months. After each procedure, the remaining skin is stretched and the incision is closed. After this heals, a little more of the scar is removed, until all that remains is a narrow line.

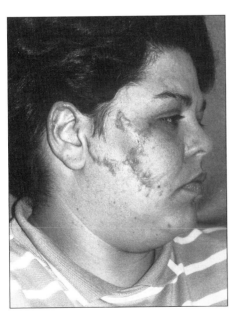 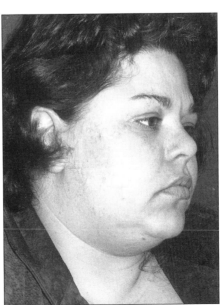

◄

*Scar revision surgery made this woman's scarring from a car accident barely noticeable.*

Steroid drugs may be injected directly into a scar to help flatten and fade it. The steroid stops the production of collagen, slowing the growth of scar tissue. Keloid or hypertrophic scars are sometimes treated in this way. Steroid injections also may be used in conjunction with other scar revision procedures in order to refine the results.

Z-plasty is a technique for releasing a contracted scar. Hit by flying glass when her car was struck by a turning vehicle, Laura developed an unsightly scar that tightened as it healed, pulling her eyelid down. The surgeon made an incision along the length of the scar, and then made little cuts above and below it at angles to form a Z. The small flaps of skin were readjusted and carefully stitched, resulting in a smoother, narrower scar that did not pull the skin.

Another technique, called the running W-plasty, was used by Shirley's surgeon to camouflage the scar on her cheek. A running W-plasty breaks up a straight-line scar into a series of tiny triangles that blend more easily into the natural skin texture. A similar technique is the geometric broken-line closure, which converts the scar into a series of tiny squares and triangles. The scar is not eliminated—in fact, it may become slightly longer—but it no longer attracts notice the way a straight line would.

Scars resulting from burns and other extensive injuries may be treated with a flap technique. Flaps are sections of healthy tissue with a blood supply. A flap may be cut loose on three sides from an adjacent area, then lifted and rotated into position to cover the damaged area. If this is not possible, a section of skin, complete with underlying tissue and blood vessels, may be taken from elsewhere in the body—such as the forearm, abdomen, or upper leg. This flap, called a free flap, is then connected to a blood supply and sutured into its new position.

Scars that have a rough or elevated appearance may be smoothed by means of skin resurfacing techniques. Often, a short-pulse carbon dioxide laser is used. This device emits powerful bursts of high-intensity light that vaporize the scar tissue with little or no damage to surrounding areas of the skin. In some cases, raised or bumpy scars may be treated with dermabrasion or chemical peeling. (See Chapter 9 for more about skin resurfacing.)

Often, more than one treatment, or a combination of techniques, is needed to attain the best results. "The doctor did dermabrasion, and several Z-plasty procedures, followed by laser abrasion," says Laura. "I still have a scar, but people don't stare at my face anymore. I can live with the way I look now."

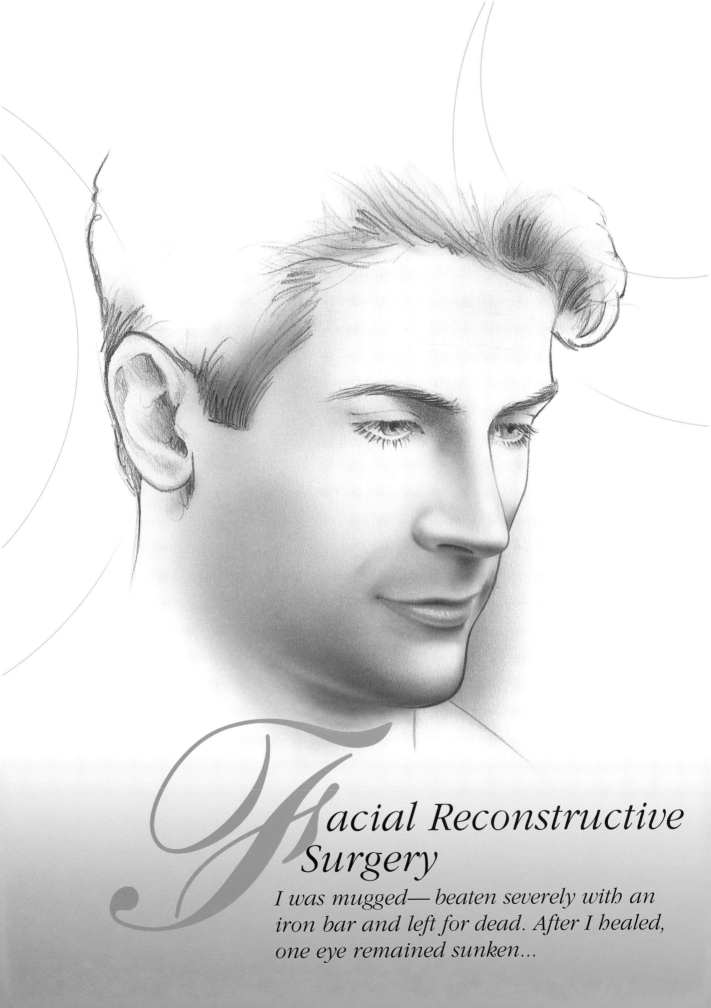

# Facial Reconstructive Surgery

*I was mugged— beaten severely with an iron bar and left for dead. After I healed, one eye remained sunken...*

# Facial Reconstructive Surgery

*"I was mugged—beaten severely with an iron bar and left for dead. After I healed, one eye remained sunken and I looked quite deformed. It was hard to get over the anger I felt. I lost my job, in part because of my appearance. Finally I found a surgeon who could put Humpty-Dumpty back together again."*

■ *Joe Cala, age 30*

Although most people who seek facial plastic surgery do so because they want to look better, some people have a much more basic need—to look normal. A facial injury, a birth defect, or cancer surgery can have a devastating impact on the appearance. Often, the function of facial structures may be compromised as well. In such cases, specialized reconstructive techniques are needed to repair functional defects and restore a more normal appearance.

Reconstructive surgery focuses on repairing muscles, cartilage, and other soft tissues as well as the skeletal structure of the face. Reconstructive procedures may be needed to correct facial problems that have resulted from:

- skin cancer and other head and neck tumors;
- motor vehicle accidents;
- injuries sustained in bicycle or motorcycle mishaps;
- serious falls or other traumatic accidents;
- violent assault;
- infections; or
- birth defects.

The goal of reconstructive surgery is to enable the patient to have normal function (in breathing and swallowing, for example) and an acceptable appearance. Because every

11

*The goal of reconstructive surgery is to enable the patient to have normal function and an acceptable appearance.*

injury or defect of the head or face is different, reconstructive procedures are highly individualized. Before developing a treatment plan, the surgeon must evaluate the size, nature, and extent of the deformity and determine the most direct way of achieving the desired result.

Often, reconstructive surgery must be done in several stages. Because it is not always possible to predict how healing will progress or how subsequent growth may affect the outcome, ongoing evaluation and follow-up are an important part of the process. Children who have had reconstructive surgery often need to be followed for years, with additional procedures performed as they grow.

> *Bailey was born with a severe cleft lip and palate, with parts of her jaw entirely missing. Her first surgery, at age four months, repaired her lip. When she was eighteen months old, one of her ribs was removed and used to fashion the missing portion of her jaw. (Part of the rib was "banked" for future bone grafts.) Although Bailey's surgery was much more extensive than a typical cleft palate repair, today she can swallow normally and she's catching up on speech development. She recently won third place in a "Cute Kids" contest. Bailey may need many additional procedures over the coming years, but she can look forward to a normal life.*

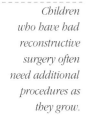

*Children who have had reconstructive surgery often need additional procedures as they grow.*

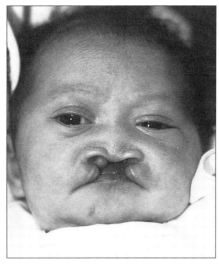
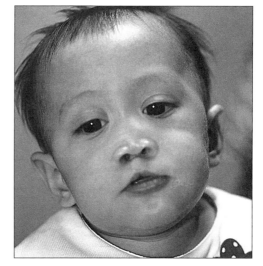

## REPAIRING SOFT TISSUES

Soft tissue repair often involves taking healthy tissue—such as skin, muscle, and connective tissue—from another part of the body and using it to replace tissue that has been damaged or destroyed.

# Reconstructive procedure restores confidence

On a bitterly cold January night, Joe Cala's life changed forever. Stopping at a gas station on his way home, he was approached by a young man who asked him for a ride home. Joe hesitated, but he took pity on the man and let him into the car. The ride turned into a nightmare as the man drew a knife and attacked Joe. After robbing him, the assailant beat Joe about the face with a metal bar and left him for dead by the side of the road.

Help arrived and Joe survived the ordeal, but—despite surgery—his face suffered terrible damage. "The bones of my face were shattered," he recalls. "There was a gaping hole in the bones under my right eye, and my eye was sunken back into my head. I really looked quite deformed." Joe had physiological problems as well, including headaches and double vision. Even worse was the emotional trauma. "They never caught the guy, and I kept seeing his face," he says. "I felt people were avoiding me because of the way I looked. I lost my job. I had a lot of anger inside."

Several months later, Joe had a reconstructive procedure that restored his appearance. "It was very high-tech," he relates. "They took a CAT scan and placed markers at particular points on my head. While operating, the surgeon could touch these markers with a special wand and a close-up view of that part of my head would be shown on a computer screen in front of him. The computer image helped him balance one side of my face with the other."

Joe's surgeon took a bone graft from the top of his head and used it to rebuild his shattered facial bones. The procedure restored Joe's eye to its proper position and improved the physical problems that had resulted from the assault. An additional procedure corrected the damage done to his nose.

"I spent only one night in the hospital after the facial reconstruction," he asserts. "Everyone was amazed at how quickly I healed."

The surgery restored Joe's confidence and helped him get over the anger he had felt. "I call on customers every day, so my appearance is very important," he says. "I'm satisfied with the way I look now, and I'm successfully running my own business. The reconstructive procedure was a big factor in helping me get on with my life."

*Skin grafts* may be used to cover wounds that cannot easily be closed directly. A skin graft is a patch of healthy skin taken from another part of the body, such as the leg or abdomen, and used to cover an area where skin is missing or damaged. Superficial injuries may be covered with a skin graft that uses only the top layers of skin. A full-thickness graft may be

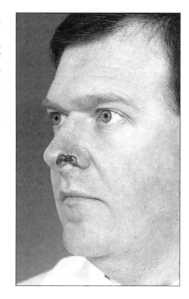 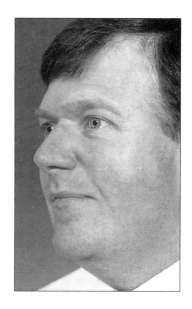

*Cheek flaps can replace nasal skin and tissue lost to cancer.*

used to close deeper wounds. If additional support is needed, a composite graft may be used. This may include skin, fat, and underlying cartilage.

*Tissue expansion* is a technique used to increase the amount of available skin to cover an injured area. A balloon-like device is inserted under healthy skin near the area to be repaired. Sterile salt water is injected into the expansion device at regular intervals over a period of weeks. This stretches the skin gradually, providing additional healthy skin that closely matches the color, sensation, and texture of the adjacent skin.

*A free flap is completely detached from the donor site, which may be the abdominal wall, the upper arm, or the leg.*

*Flap surgery* may be performed to restore form and function to areas of the face that have lost skin, fat, muscle, and even skeletal support. Flaps are sections of living tissue carrying their own blood supply that are moved from one area of the body to another. A local flap is one taken from an area adjacent to the wound. The flap remains attached at one end so that it continues to be nourished by its original blood supply. A free flap is completely detached from the donor site, which may be the abdominal wall, the upper arm, or the leg. Advanced microsurgery techniques are used to fix the flap in the new location, connecting the blood vessels and nerves of the flap to others found in the neck.

> *When a tumor attacked Ravi's face, it destroyed much of the skin and cartilage of her nose. Her nose was rebuilt using cartilage from her ear and rib. To cover the rebuilt nose, the surgeon used a flap taken from her forehead. The tumor gone, Ravi now has normal nasal function and an acceptable appearance.*

## CORRECTING STRUCTURAL ABNORMALITIES

When disease, injury, or a birth defect affects the skeletal structure of the face, reconstructive efforts must focus on providing a framework to support the soft tissues.

Surgeons use a variety of techniques, depending on the specific needs of the patient. For example, areas that appear sunken may be built up by means of implants made of a surgical-grade synthetic material. Sometimes, cheek implants (similar to those described in Chapter 6) are used to build up depressed areas in the midface.

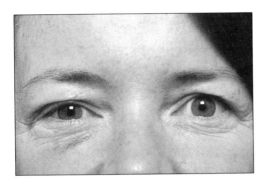 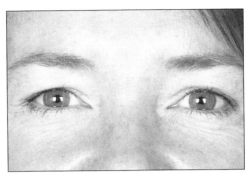

◄

*When struck in the eye playing basketball, this woman suffered double vision and a sunken eye. Reconstructive surgery improved both function and appearance.*

Serious structural deficiencies also may be corrected through the use synthetic materials that can remain safely in the body for an indefinite period. For example, a surgical-grade synthetic material may be used to provide support for the nose or other facial structures.

Broken or shattered facial bones are sometimes repaired by attaching wires to tiny screws placed in healthy bone, or by fixing metal rods or plates over the fracture. Where bone is missing or damaged beyond repair, bone may be taken from the skull, hip, or leg and grafted into place. Some types of flaps may even include bone, as well as muscle, skin, and other soft tissue.

*An accidental bump while playing with his two-year-old child shattered John M.'s cheekbone — and revealed the presence of a rare cancer that had been quietly growing inside his face. After surgery to remove the tumor, John needed several procedures to rebuild his face. First, a bone graft was done, then the surgeon inserted a large cheek implant to fill out his hollowed cheek. A flap was taken from the inside of John's upper arm to patch the hole in his face, and dermabrasion subsequently improved the appearance of the scar and evened out the difference in pigmentation between the arm and facial skin. Because the tumor affected John's ability to move his right eyelid, his surgeon implanted a tiny gold weight that helps him close the eye naturally. John is glad to be alive — and satisfied with his appearance as well.*

# *Facial reanimation surgery*

Imagine the tragedy of not being able to smile or use your eyes expressively. Sometimes an injury or medical condition leaves a person with a face that is partially paralyzed, resulting in a drooping eye, a mouth that sags on one side, or a cheek that appears to have fallen in.

Specialized facial plastic surgery techniques can improve some types of facial paralysis and restore normal appearance and function.

In a normal face, the muscles on either side exert tension on each other to keep the features in balance. When paralysis on one side occurs, the normal side is also affected, because the "pull" from the other side is no longer there. Damage to certain nerves may cause drooping of an eye or the corner of the mouth when the face is at rest. In some cases, certain types of movement—such as the ability to close the eyes—may be inhibited.

To improve distortion caused by facial paralysis, an incision similar to the one used for a facelift is made to expose the support structures of the face. A strip of supportive tissue—called fascia—may be removed and used to create a sling to support a drooping lip or eye. Muscles and fascia can be lifted and tightened or moved to a new location to exert tension where it is needed.

Special implants, customized for the patient's face, are used in some cases to fill a depression where muscle tissue has atrophied or has been removed. A tiny gold weight—smaller than a pinkie fingernail—may be implanted in an eyelid to enable it to close. Surgeons can even take a ligament from the leg or elsewhere and use it to make a sling to support certain structures.

To restore function to paralyzed facial features, a procedure called a free muscle transfer may be used. Muscle and nerve tissue is taken from another part of the body, such as the chest wall, and used to replace damaged facial tissue. The muscles are attached in their new location and the nerve is connected to a branch of the facial nerve. Healing takes several months, but most patients eventually notice significant improvement of their facial function.

Although facial paralysis can be emotionally devastating, modern facial plastic surgery techniques can go a long way toward restoring normal appearance and function in patients with damaged facial nerves.

*Where bone is missing or damaged beyond repair, bone may be taken from the skull, hip, or leg and grafted into place.*

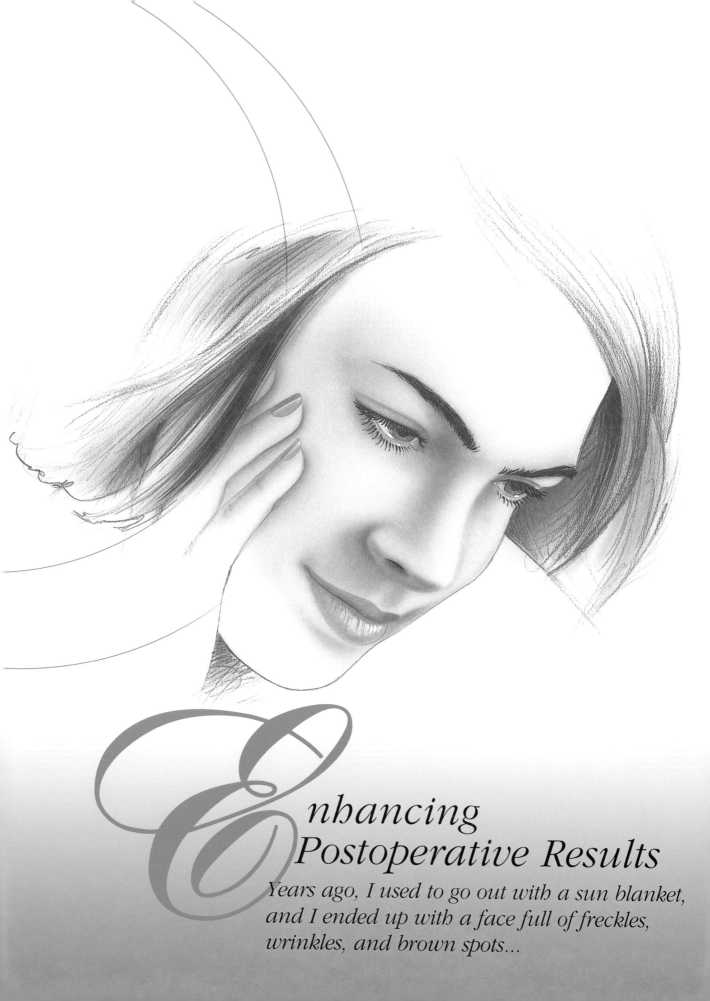

# Enhancing Postoperative Results

*Years ago, I used to go out with a sun blanket, and I ended up with a face full of freckles, wrinkles, and brown spots...*

# Enhancing Postoperative Results

*"Years ago, I used to go out with a sun blanket, and I ended up with a face full of freckles, wrinkles, and brown spots. Facial plastic surgery restored my skin beautifully, and now I practice preventive maintenance. I avoid the sun, and I'm careful to cleanse and moisturize my face daily. I want my lovely new skin to last."*

■ *Ronnie Lazar, age 72*

If you plan to have facial plastic surgery, the best time to begin thinking of your postoperative care regimen is before you have the procedure. In fact, there are a number of things you can do ahead of time to prepare yourself for facial plastic surgery both physically and emotionally. Advance preparation also can enhance your surgical result.

After the procedure, you should follow your surgeon's instructions meticulously. This is a time to pamper yourself. Many facial plastic surgery patients feel a bit of a letdown after the procedure. This is only natural. The final results are not yet visible, your face may be bruised or swollen, and you may feel somewhat drained from the surgery. Give yourself time to heal—and focus on the compliments you'll receive when you unveil the fresh, new you.

"After my facelift, I felt isolated and depressed," recalls Karen A. "My face was swollen, and I was afraid I'd never look like myself again." Karen took comfort in her surgeon's assurance that her feelings were not unusual and her healing was progressing satisfactorily. Within a few days, she was feeling her cheerful self again, and two months after the procedure she was able to declare jubilantly, "My face is still improving, but already I look fabulous. This is the best thing I've ever done!"

12

*An appointment with an image consultant shortly after your surgery can give you a real psychological boost.*

## PLAN AHEAD TO BEAT THE "POST-OP BLUES"

A little bit of advance planning can help you beat the "post-op blues." Says Julie W., "I knew I'd be staying in, so I prepared myself for it. I made sure I had a supply of good books and videos in the house, and I arranged to get help with housework so I wouldn't have to do anything I didn't want to do."

It's important to plan enough time for your recovery. "I followed my surgeon's instructions to the letter," Karen explains. "Carrying out my skin care regimen gave me something to focus on, and I'm convinced it made a big difference in the results as well."

An appointment with an image consultant shortly after your surgery can give you a real psychological boost. In fact, some facial plastic surgeons even have an image specialist on staff to consult with postoperative patients. A professional beauty consultation can lift your spirits, speed the healing process, and help you to put your best face forward.

If you would rather not have friends and co-workers know that you are having surgery, you may want to schedule a beauty makeover a week or so before surgery. A dramatic change in your hairstyle just before you have a procedure can help divert attention away from your face and make the results of the surgery less obvious. Go from curly to straight—or vice versa. Add subtle highlights to your hair color. Try a bold new haircut or adopt an upswept style (with a soft fringe of bangs to cover facelift incisions).

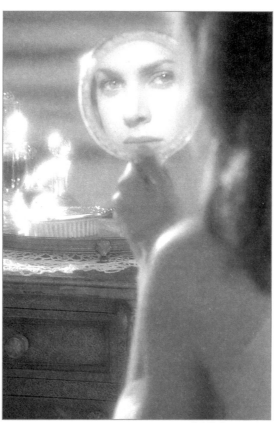

©1996, Comstock, Inc.

Updated makeup and careful use of color can disguise any swelling or bruising that occurs. Accessories—such as an eye-catching bracelet or lapel pin—are another way to draw the focus away from your face. You may find friends saying, "You look so well rested after your vacation!" rather than "Oh, did you have your face done?"

Most importantly, prepare yourself emotionally for the procedure. "My surgeon made it clear that the day after the facelift I would look like I had been in a train wreck—and he was right!" Karen laughs. "I loved his honesty. It helped me to stay on an even keel afterward. Although I felt weepy, I knew it was a temporary thing and I just needed to hang on. In a few days, I was looking better than ever and feeling great again."

Here are some tips that may help your recovery go smoothly:

- Before the surgery, prepare and freeze a number of tasty, nutritious meals. This way you can take it easy for a few days, but still get a good diet.

- Ask your surgeon about any postoperative dietary limitations. For example, if you are having surgery on your jaw, cheeks, or chin, you may want to lay in a supply of nourishing foods that don't require much chewing—like yogurt, applesauce, pudding, soup, and macaroni.

- Clean your home thoroughly just before surgery. This can help minimize exposure to infection-causing germs—and enable you to avoid unnecessary household chores during the early healing period.

- Get the prescriptions for any medications you may need after surgery and have them filled ahead of time.

- Line up your support system. You'll need someone to drive you home after surgery. You also may want a family member or a close friend nearby for a few days to help with your postoperative care and provide encouragement during the healing period.

- Plan your wardrobe for the day of surgery and the week or so afterward. Choose loose, comfortable clothing that opens down the front, so you won't need to pull anything over your head.

Finally, relax! Plan to pamper yourself a little. A positive mental outlook can actually speed healing and help you look and feel your best.

## CHECK YOUR DIET—BEFORE AND AFTER SURGERY

Good nutrition is an important part of preparing for facial plastic surgery. What you eat affects both the surface of your skin and the underlying structures, including nerves, blood vessels, cartilage, and muscle tissues. A healthy diet promotes a vibrant complexion and an overall healthy glow. It also helps ensure that you have the inner resources to heal quickly and resume your active lifestyle. That's why it's a good idea to pay particular attention to your diet before having facial plastic surgery. After a facial plastic surgery procedure, good nutritional habits can help keep your new appearance looking fresh for as long as possible.

In general, a healthy diet is one that includes plenty of fresh fruits and vegetables, complex carbohydrates such as bread, cereal, and pasta (whole grains in particular), lean meat (or a protein substitute), and low-fat dairy foods. Don't embark on any type of severely restrictive diet in the month before surgery. If you need to lose weight, take it off slowly by reducing your caloric intake and increasing your activity level. Vegetarians need to be particularly careful to maintain adequate levels of the amino acids essential to wound healing. If you are a vegetarian, discuss your diet with the surgeon well in advance.

A balanced diet can help ensure that you are getting adequate supplies of the nutrients that promote optimal healing. Vitamin C, for example, is necessary for the production of collagen, the connective tissue that supports the skin. Vitamin K speeds blood clotting. If your

*A balanced diet can help ensure that you are getting adequate supplies of the nutrients that promote optimal healing.*

eating habits have not been ideal, you might want to discuss your concerns with your surgeon. In some cases, a supplement may be recommended.

Don't take any nutritional supplements without informing your doctor, however. In fact, you should discuss all medications you are taking with your doctor well in advance of surgery. Certain nutritional supplements—such as vitamin E and selenium—may delay clotting time and increase the amount of blood loss. Some medications, including over-the-counter analgesics and anti-inflammatory drugs, also may have an adverse effect. Your surgeon may advise you to discontinue certain nutritional supplements and medications for a time before and after surgery.

---

## Smoking can affect surgical results

If you're planning a facial plastic surgery procedure, be sure to discuss your smoking habits openly with your surgeon. Because cigarette smoking affects the blood supply to the skin, it may slow healing time and increase the risk of bleeding and other complications. Although smoking will not necessarily prevent you from having surgery, your doctor should be made aware of any factor that may affect your surgical results.

In some cases, possible problems may be forestalled by modifying the procedure slightly. For example, the length and placement of the incisions may be adapted or a specific medication may be recommended. More likely, your surgeon may want you to quit smoking for several weeks before and after the surgery. This vital step can help give you the best surgical results possible and speed up your healing time. Follow your doctor's instructions carefully.

You may want to consider cutting down on smoking or even eliminating it entirely. It is well documented that smoking contributes to the formation of facial wrinkles, particularly around the mouth. Cutting back can help to preserve the benefits of your facial plastic surgery procedure by delaying the formation of new wrinkles. In fact, if you are a smoker, quitting is one of the most effective steps you can take toward slowing the aging process and maintaining the health and beauty of your skin.

---

## GIVE YOURSELF TIME TO HEAL

Your surgery is over, the swelling is down, and you're feeling great. Can you get right back to your regular routine?

Before jumping right in, think about whether your everyday activities will interfere in any way with your continued healing. You should plan on taking it easy for at least the first two weeks after surgery. Protect your incisions, rest when you feel tired, eat foods that do not require strenuous chewing, and avoid arguments or emotional extremes that may put strain on your incisions.

Sleep with your head elevated during the first two weeks—and sleep alone to avoid being accidentally bumped by a sleeping partner. Avoid bending over, picking up small children, and lifting anything heavy— actions that may aggravate swelling and precipitate bleeding. If you have had a facelift or neck surgery, do not turn your head from side to side—rotate your entire upper body instead.

You may feel great, but be careful not to get back into your regular fitness routine too soon after having facial plastic surgery. Vigorous exercise elevates your blood pressure, which can cause swelling and interfere with healing. On the other hand,

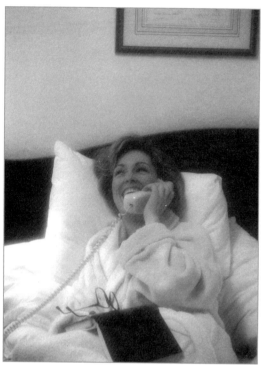

©1997, Comstock, Inc.

moderate exercise is a good idea. Gentle physical activity can give you a psychological boost, encourage good blood circulation, and speed the healing process.

In general, you should avoid strenuous workouts for four to six weeks after surgery. Concentrate instead on gentle stretches and calisthenics for the first few weeks after your incisions have healed. Avoid floor work and exercises that involve resistance or that cause your head to drop below your waist, as these types of movements may raise the blood pressure and put a strain on your incisions. Be sure to avoid any sort of activity that can cause an inadvertent blow to the face. Swimming is fine exercise beginning about three weeks after surgery, but do not dive for at least six to eight weeks.

Get your doctor's advice before resuming any vigorous exercise routine. Then start slowly, and intensify your exercise routine gradually after healing is complete.

## USING COSMETICS AFTER SURGERY

How soon you can apply cosmetics after surgery will depend on the procedures you have had. Generally, cosmetics may be applied as soon as the incisions have healed—usually about a week after surgery. If you have had a skin resurfacing procedure, you may need to wait a little longer. Follow your doctor's advice.

You may want to use specially formulated cosmetics that are available for facial plastic surgery patients. High-coverage corrective cosmetics are available for both men and women to camouflage scars, bruises, and excess redness. Even if you don't need a high-coverage

*Updated makeup and careful use of color can disguise any swelling or bruising that occurs.*

product, it's a good idea to select cosmetics that are extra gentle and easily removable if irritation does occur. Products containing fragrance or alcohol should be avoided during the first few weeks.

Cleanse your skin carefully, following your doctor's instructions. Surgery may temporarily make dry skin more dry and oily skin more oily. If your skin is dry or oily, ask your surgeon about using a gentle moisturizer or astringent. Be sure that everything that comes in contact with your face is completely sanitary. Use cotton swabs, cotton balls, and disposable sponges instead of cosmetic brushes. Apply cosmetics gently to avoid pulling the skin.

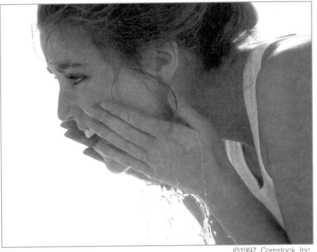

©1997, Comstock, Inc.

*To neutralize discoloration, apply a small amount of neutralizer in the opposite tone— green to correct excess redness, yellow to conceal purple bruises, and purple to cover yellow discoloration.*

 Keep your makeup simple. Forget bold colors that may draw attention to your scars and go for a more muted, natural look. If discoloration is evident, use a neutralizing toner before applying your foundation. Underbase toners are available in green, yellow, and purple. To neutralize discoloration, apply a small amount of neutralizer in the opposite tone—green to correct excess redness, yellow to conceal purple bruises, and purple to cover yellow discoloration. Then sponge on a high-coverage or regular foundation that matches your natural skin tone and blend carefully. A translucent powder helps set the foundation and yields a soft, natural look.

# *Make sunscreen a part of daily facial care*

Applying a sunscreen should be part of your every day facial care routine, particularly after you've had facial plastic surgery. The sun's ultraviolet radiation is extremely damaging to the skin. Not only does it cause genetic mutations in skin cells that may lead to cancer, it also speeds the aging process, leading to premature wrinkles and age spots.

After facial plastic surgery, your skin is especially sensitive to the sun. If you have had a skin resurfacing procedure, sun exposure may cause pigment changes, leading to blotchiness or variations in skin tone. Plan to protect yourself from the sun for at least the first six months after surgery, by wearing a wide-brimmed hat and sunglasses and staying in the shade whenever possible.

Apply a sunscreen to your face any time you plan to be outside for any length of time. Use a broad-spectrum product that offers an SPF of 15 or higher. To get the most from your sunscreen, be sure to apply it properly. To shield you from ultraviolet radiation effectively, the product must stay on the surface of your skin. Do not rub it in, but smooth it on with a light touch, just as you would foundation makeup.

# More Patient Information from the AAFPRS

## The AAFPRS Patient Brochure Series

Single copies of the following brochures are available free to patients who call the AAFPRS's toll-free number: 1-800-332-FACE. The brochures contain information about the most common facial plastic and reconstructive procedures in use today:

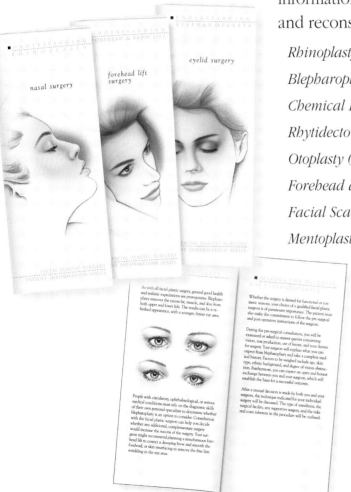

*Rhinoplasty (nasal surgery)\**

*Blepharoplasty (eyelid surgery)\**

*Chemical Peel and Dermabrasion*

*Rhytidectomy (facelift surgery)\**

*Otoplasty (ear surgery)*

*Forehead and Brow Lift*

*Facial Scar Revision*

*Mentoplasty (chin surgery)*

*Laser Surgery*

*Hair Replacement*

*What Is a Facial Plastic Surgeon?*

*\* Also available in Spanish*

# Facial Plastic Surgery Today

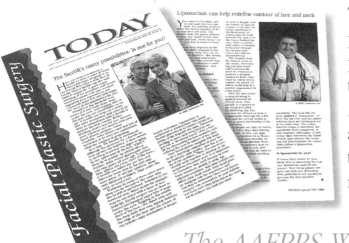

The AAFPRS produces a quarterly patient education newsletter that will provide you with up-to-date information about facial plastic surgery. *Facial Plastic Surgery Today* is on-line at the AAFPRS web site or available through the Academy's toll-free number: 1-800-332-FACE.

# The AAFPRS Web Site

Visit the AAFPRS web site and you will find the latest information about the major facial plastic surgery procedures in use today, including new techniques such as laser resurfacing, an introduction to the AAFPRS and its programs and patient publications, and the names and phone numbers of facial plastic surgeons in other cities. The Academy's web address is *http://www.facemd.org.*

# AAFPRS Information Service

The Academy's toll-free number, 1-800-332-FACE, gives patients access to the latest information on facial plastic surgery procedures as well as a listing of qualified facial plastic surgeons in other locations.

# The Face Book: A Consumer's Guide to Facial Plastic Surgery

Additional copies of *The Face Book* can be ordered by calling 1-800-332-FACE.

# About the American Academy of Facial Plastic and Reconstructive Surgery

Founded in 1964, the American Academy of Facial Plastic and Reconstructive Surgery—with 2,700 members—is the world's largest association of facial plastic surgeons and the only organization dedicated solely to the advancement of the highest quality of facial plastic and reconstructive surgery.

To achieve its mission, the AAFPRS:

- Ascribes to rigorous professional standards;

- Offers a widely recognized program of postresidency education;

- Disseminates information that assures recognition of specialty standards among professional medical organizations, healthcare providers, legislative and regulatory bodies, and the public;

- Supports the concept that facial plastic surgery requires intensive training and competence, embodies high ethical standards, artistic ideals, commitment to humanitarian service, and a desire to enhance the quality of human life; and

- Assists members with practice management, to assure the delivery of high quality, cost-effective medicine and surgery.

Long recognized by the American Medical Association as a national medical specialty society representing facial plastic surgery, the AAFPRS holds an official seat in the AMA House of Delegates and on the American College of Surgeons Board of Governors.

The majority of AAFPRS members and fellows are certified by the American Board of Otolaryngology, which includes examination in facial plastic and reconstructive surgery. Other AAFPRS members are surgeons certified in ophthalmology, plastic surgery, and dermatology. Some members additionally are diplomates of the American Board of Facial Plastic and Reconstructive Surgery.

# ACKNOWLEDGMENTS

Since 1988, when the American Academy of Facial Plastic and Reconstructive Surgery (AAFPRS) published the first edition of *The Face Book,* hundreds of readers—patients and surgeons alike—have contacted the AAFPRS. Most commented on how helpful the book was to patients who were considering facial plastic surgery. More recently, others have suggested ways the book might be updated to make it even more valuable. After all, they point out, the last 10 years have seen major advances in surgical techniques, and people like to know what's new and how it might affect them.

To all of these readers, we express thanks for the positive feedback and constructive criticism. Your response to the original *Face Book* led to the appointment one year ago of a special editorial board to guide the development of a new edition of the book. Since then, members of this board have devoted countless hours to determining the scope of the new book and ensuring that their vision was carried out in each word and image chosen. We gratefully acknowledge the contributions of this board, including its chairman, Wm. Russell Ries, MD, and these members: Becky L. McGraw-Wall, MD; David Reiter, MD, DMD; William W. Shockley, MD; and Robert L. Simons, MD.

For sharing their medical knowledge through in-depth interviews, organizing patient interviews, and reviewing manuscript, we also thank: Shan R. Baker, MD; Ferdinand F. Becker, MD; William J. Binder, MD; Kenneth A. Buchwach, MD; Paul J. Carniol, MD; Jeffrey J. Colton, MD; Ted A. Cook, MD; Steven M. Denenberg, MD; Wallace K. Dyer II, MD; Jim L. English, MD; Richard W. Fleming, MD; John L. Frodel Jr., MD; Linda Gage-White, MD; Julio F. Gallo, MD; Jim E. Gilmore, MD; Michael S. Godin, MD; Calvin M. Johnson Jr., MD; Frank M. Kamer, MD; Raymond J. Konior, MD; Wayne F. Larrabee Jr., MD; William H. Lindsey, MD; Devinder S. Mangat, MD; Toby G. Mayer, MD; Gary J. Nishioka, MD; Ira D. Papel, MD; Norman J. Pastorek, MD; Stephen W. Perkins, MD; Vito C. Quatela, MD; Daniel E. Rousso, MD; Sigmund L. Sattenspiel, MD; Larry D. Schoenrock, MD; J. George Smith Jr., MD; Jon F. Strohmeyer, MD; J. Regan Thomas, MD; Tom D. Wang, MD; and J. Michael Willett, MD.

Additionally, thanks go to S. Randolph Waldman, MD, who as AAFPRS vice president for public affairs, helped to see that the book meets a variety of public information needs. In this same vein, we appreciate the contributions of Stephen C. Duffy, AAFPRS executive vice president, and Rita C. Magness, AAFPRS publications and marketing director, who directed necessary resources to the project and oversaw its progress, budget, and timely delivery.

We owe a special debt to the patients who recounted their experiences. Most people who have had facial plastic surgery are happy to talk about it. In most cases, the patients' own names have been used with their permission. In some cases, the names have been changed to protect confidentiality. In some other cases, to avoid any intrusion into privacy, the facts of several surgeries have been combined into a description that, the AAFPRS believes, accurately reflects typical experiences.

Finally, but certainly not least, we extend special thanks to the editorial team at Network Communications, especially T. Susan Hill, who served as executive editor of *The Face Book;* Angela Martin, senior medical editor; and Sharon L. Cool, production editor; and also to Tony Magliano, managing partner of Strata-G Communications, Inc., who served as the book's senior designer and medical illustrator, and Gwene Daugherty and Kelly Pennington, also with Strata-G Communications. Most of these people worked on the original *Face Book* or the Academy's patient brochures and patient education newsletter, and we are fortunate that they continue to translate our medial science into informative and readable prose.

We hope this book gives you some understanding of the untiring dedication of AAFPRS members to making the highest possible quality of facial plastic surgery available to the public.

Peter A. Adamson, MD
*President, American Academy of Facial Plastic and Reconstructive Surgery*
*1996–1997*